Hypn

By the same author:

Self-Hypnosis

Hypnosex

Pleasure control – the amazing new way to improve your love life, enhance your relationships and enjoy greater sexual fulfilment through self-hypnosis

Valerie Austin

Thorsons
An Imprint of HarperCollinsPublishers

Thorsons
An Imprint of HarperCollins*Publishers*
77–85 Fulham Palace Road
Hammersmith, London W6 8JB

1160 Battery Street
San Francisco, California 94111–1213

Published by Thorsons 1996

10 9 8 7 6 5 4 3 2 1

A catalogue record for this book
is available from the British Library

ISBN 0 7225 3335 7

Printed and bound in Great Britain by
Caledonian International Book Manufacturing Ltd, Glasgow

Dedication

To my husband – wherever he is

Contents

Acknowledgements

United Kingdom, my home:
Roy Stockdill, my agent and friend, for his constant
encouragement and occasional bullying.
Cynthia Payne, Philip Hodson and Adam Cole ... three
people who are all experts on sex in their respective fields
and who gave me valuable insights.
Professor G. Lucas, Keeper of the Herbarium at Kew
Gardens.
David Attenborough and his masterful book on plants.

Special helpers in my research...
Pierre Marcar, a man of many talents, for his superbly
descriptive suggestions.
My many students, especially Deborah Marshall-Warren,
an excellent example.
Ricky and his Magician Course.
Nicholas, head chef at Stringfellow's; whenever I need
a menu for one of my books, I call him.
Duncan McCall, a lovely gentleman hypnotherapist.
All my clients.
And last, but certainly not least, Uri Geller for his fantastic
skills.

Malaysia, a country that taught me so much:
His Honourable Dato Lee Kim Sei, Minister of Health, for his acceptance and support in presenting my diplomas for hypnotherapy training.
Professor Dato Dr Abdul Halim Othman, Dean of the University of Kebangsaan, for his recognition, trust and for giving me the honour of addressing his students of psychology through the years.
Malaysia Airlines, for the best landings and service I have ever experienced; being a pilot myself, I tend automatically to 'round out' as the plane lands.
Malaysia Tourist Board for their valued help.
My special students in paradise: Irshad, Jürgen, Molly and Tom.
Mavis and Azman for allowing me to consult in paradise at the Holiday Villa, Langkawi, and Holiday Inn on the Park.
Leo Cusher for placing me at the top of the world in the Crown Princess.
Palangi Beach Resort, Langkawi, for allowing me to feel like a Prime Minister in the suite that was specially built for *her* visit in 1989.
Datai resort, Langkawi, a marvellous venue for my courses, and Irshad for the wonderful treks in those 5,000 private acres of rain forest that taught me how close our human strategies are to those of nature.
My special friend Siti Baizura, a lady who has her name written on the moon.
Haji Ayub, my mischievous minder.
Ike Ong, who gave me my legends.
Mohd Yuzer Mohd Yusoff, for his truly golden holidays, creating a perfect experience for my 'Learning in Paradise', a business colleague and valued friend.
Prince Tommy and Paul, a spiritual light.

ACKNOWLEDGEMENTS

All my friends and clients in Malaysia for a peek into a true paradise.
And, of course, Dr Lau.

USA:
Frank Dana, a true Hollywood hypnotherapist with a big heart; my many US hypnotherapy friends, especially Jade who suffered an even worse memory loss than me; and all my friends in the film industry.
Gil Boyne, for his confidence in hypnotherapy and beginning the cure for my memory, so that I can live happily.

Tonga
Haniteli, Director of the Ministry of Agriculture; Papiloa Foiake from the Friendly Islands; my friends in Tonga.

Finally ...
A special 'thank you' to Kay Keirnan of the Bluestone Clinic, a grand lady and miracle worker, for keeping my back from pain and for her PEME machine which cured my physical ailments.

Introduction

Wonderful, uninhibited sex is everybody's right,
so clear your mind for it

It is everybody's right as a human being to enjoy the wonders
of the body. So why should others have the most incredible
sexual experiences and not you? You can have them too! Or,
if you have them already, you can have better ones. This
book is intended to help you to free yourself of restrictive,
old, incorrect mind programming, leaving you free to
explore the incredible journey into sexual ecstasy. If you
clear your mind of unproductive inhibitions, it can instruct
the body for wonderful sexual pleasure – erotic heights that
are in balance and correct with your being.

Hypnosis is a safe way to help you do this and enjoy a
sexual relationship – safe because you yourself are at the
controls and because there is no danger of your mind being
changed if, in so doing, it would cause you conflict that
would be detrimental to your life in general.

The book is divided into five chapters, forming a complete
do-it-yourself guide on how to use trance and hypnosis to
reach the parts that are not already achieving ecstasy beyond
belief. It is written for:

• The person who wants to increase their sexual pleasures,
even though they may be adequate already. However

wonderful a relationship may be, there is always room for improvement! Knowledge provides the tools to enhance an already happy relationship.

- The person who is having a problem attaining sexual joy, for whatever reason, whether a feeling of inadequacy, lack of self-esteem, ignorance, an unhappy experience, fear of homosexuality or lesbian tendencies, or the fear of being hurt emotionally.
- The person who has never enjoyed the pleasures of full sexual fulfilment, perhaps because their first and only lover was their spouse or partner, whom they may love dearly and do not want to leave but are no longer sexually attracted to. Their circumstances may not be likely to change, but their dissatisfaction can certainly be directed into a more fulfilling sexual harmony.
- Couples who want to work together on their relationship, eliminating their inhibitions and bringing about greater sexual kinship.
- Couples who want to rekindle their relationship, fall in love again and reawaken those faded, exotic experiences of when they first fell in love.

Although this book has not been written to be salacious or prurient, occasionally I have found it necessary to be explicit. I have also drawn freely on my own relationship experiences – some of them good, some disastrous!

THE BRAIN IS THE MOST EROTIC ORGAN IN THE BODY

This is precisely where it starts: the instruction from the brain to the sensory system. All the brain's electrical responses are gathered from a variety of informative senses. Vision, smell, taste, hearing, touch – all play an important role in the sophisticated and delicate natural act of procreation. The incredible pleasure when mind and body are in tune is nature's way of temptation to make babies. If sex weren't so lustful and exciting, the human race would be in deep trouble. So why do we have so many hang-ups about it and, more importantly, can we do anything to correct the kind of unwanted sexual behaviour that interrupts our pleasure or spoils our relationships?

The following pages are designed to help you develop yourself, so you have complete pleasure control. As already mentioned, you may feel that you are sexually satisfied and do not need any help. But any skill is always capable of being developed and that includes love-making. Alternatively, you may feel that your problems have too strong a hold for you to ever be able to do anything about them. I can assure you that however serious you feel your problems are, you can make the change just by making up your mind to. Once you have made the commitment, then all you need is a little practice and some simple self-hypnosis. The pay-off is complete sexual fulfilment!

These days, it is considered quite common and even fashionable to see a counsellor or therapist for a relationship problem, although the problem may be the scapegoat for a sexual dilemma that has not been dealt with – a dilemma that one or both of the parties has not yet acknowledged, not allowed to be aired. There are a whole range of fears that may have delayed a discussion on the subject. The most popular excuse is the fear of hurting your partner – which is probably quite accurate. However, keeping silent about a problem just suppresses it and ultimately will only make things worse.

If no help is sought or the problem not aired, the next step is silent acceptance. The problem becomes something the respective partners are prepared to thrust into the background on an 'out of sight, out of mind' basis. The danger comes when one partner becomes vulnerable and is attracted to someone else. 'My wife/husband doesn't understand me' will ultimately be the justification for this infidelity. This is probably the oldest cliché in 'The Adulterer's Handbook' but it's often correct, however unfair. But it does take two to argue or, indeed, to cover up a problem. If you are having problems communicating with your lover, their body language will give you all the signs you need and hypnosis can alert your senses so you pick up those all-important tell-tale signals.

There may also be a definite breakdown in the communication between your own thoughts and actions, resulting in a bad performance. If the mind is programmed incorrectly, then it may divorce itself from the physical body, resulting in unwanted behaviour and malfunction. Finding the source and correcting it is where hypnosis can win – problem solved.

An example of when communication can break down is where an artificial state of sexual excitement is induced. Many users of drugs like Ecstasy and cocaine find this out to their dismay. For instance, Ecstasy can give the impression that you are sexually aroused but it does not always link up physically with the sexual organs, resulting in one of the partners not being able to perform. In the man it is more obvious, simply because he either doesn't get an erection or loses it before the actual sexual intercourse. Because he may believe he is showing a weakness, a fear of non-performance may then creep in, the dreaded 'performance anxiety', while the woman may just lose interest and end up having to play-act. Every woman seems to be a master (or should that be 'mistress'?!) at acting this specialized role at any time, any place. If they wish, women can perform a magnificent non-existent climax. Many men are absolutely sure that they can tell whether their partner is play-acting – but the wives' story is different.

An orgasm is a 'chemical reaction.' So communication between the thought and the action of love-making can also be seriously impaired if there has been interference due to artificial, physical or trauma-related experiences. Thus, even though there may have not been any artificial stimulants, the male feels excited. But what follows can be a variety of complications, from premature ejaculation to other serious sexual dysfunctions. And although the woman never needs to worry about premature ejaculation, she may be going through a similar experience in her mind, also resulting in a problem.

Many misguided ideas have been passed down to us, such as that the way to satisfy a women is to spend hours of love-making in foreplay before a climax, when in reality the amount of time needed is very flexible, depending on the woman's own beliefs and preferences. If the man is oblivious to how important timing is and puts his full energy into prolonging the love-making before orgasm, it can become a nightmare to the woman instead of a pleasure. The unfortunate part is, she cannot tell him in case his reaction is to blame her.

Another annoyance to many women is the common male obsession that size is important. So many men think that a massive appendage will turn all women on, and the more obscenely big it is, the more a woman likes it. This is a common belief amongst editors of national newspapers, judging by some of the stories they publish! All I can suggest is to use a little common sense. It can get very tedious for a woman to have to keep on explaining that there is a limit.

A related problem is that some men find it rather alarming

that many women will tell all to their special friends, detailing the man's performance. This does not include all women, but we are talking about human nature here and that's not going to change. However, genuine lovers with a completely fulfilling sexual relationship will have no problem issues to discuss, so privacy is more likely.

Most sexual problems stem from the lack of communication between thought and reality, or presumptions by the over-confident and the misreading of pertinent signs – definitely not a good basis for a caring relationship. However, a simple instruction in hypnosis can correct this unthinking behaviour. By bringing each partner's attention to detail, you should be able to 'read' your lover, resulting in a connected sexual harmony.

ONE

'The men who give you the best sex are the ones who also give you nervous breakdowns'
CYNTHIA PAYNE

Why is this book called *Hypnosex*? Because it is designed as a positive approach to guide you to achieve fulfilment and freedom, sexually, with the partner of your choice, using hypnosis to help you reach this goal. It also includes techniques to help you attract a compatible, or more compatible, partner, if you are not already in a relationship or feel you are in the wrong one. An alternative title could be 'Sex in Trance', because later I shall be showing you how you can use the trance state to improve your love life.

The reasons for reading this book are several and varied. As already mentioned, it may be that you want to increase satisfaction in your already pleasurable love life, or perhaps achieve a sexual satisfaction that has eluded you; it could be because of a confidence problem; you might have married for money and find sex disappointing or even an ordeal; you may have a sexual preference that is not acceptable to your partner; you may have stopped fancying your partner, or never fancied them sexually in the first place, although you feel you love them. This book is geared both for the person who finds it difficult to enjoy the basic human pleasure of an incredible sexual experience and for those individuals or couples who wish to increase their already satisfactory sex life.

I am presuming that love still plays a major role in your scenario, hence your search for greater satisfaction. Otherwise, the hypnotic suggestions I shall be showing you how to construct may be jeopardized, simply because the relationship you are trying to rekindle could be bad for you. If this is the case – and if so, you are more than likely already fully aware of it – then you can use this book to help you move on, as I did, and then reprogramme yourself to attract the *right* person. Fortunately, most relationships are capable of being rescued ... that is, if you want them to be.

The fact that you have read even this far indicates that you have a mind open for improvement. I'm sure you will find some very interesting and useful new approaches to reprogramming your mind, allowing you to achieve longer, better and more frequent sexual pleasure than you could ever have dreamed possible.

My research was extensive. I interviewed psychologists, psychiatrists, sex therapists, general practitioners, even a Royal doctor who supplements his income by treating very highly paid hookers! I spoke to romantic novelists, Fleet Street journalists, agony aunts, celebrity hairdressers privy to secrets of the rich and famous, people who buy, or get paid for, sex, and a range of men and women with unusual sexual preferences.

Britain's best known brothel keeper, the legendary Cynthia Payne, 'Madam Sin', created a business out of catering for men with unusual sexual preferences, achieving fame with her notorious luncheon voucher sex parties. The film *Personal Services*, starring Julie Walters, was based on her life and now there is also the video, aptly called *The House of Cyn*. Cynthia catered for gentlemen over 50, with reductions for pensioners. Many of these men had been sexually abandoned by their wives, who were usually totally unaware that their husbands had looked elsewhere for satisfaction, foolishly imagining they were happy enough at home.

'Take it from me, the men who give you the best sex are the ones who also give you nervous breakdowns,' says Cynthia. A cynical comment, perhaps, but many women will no doubt know what she means! It might be wise to note that many of the men who visited her parties started out on their marriages with what they believed to be the love of all time. One partner, or sometimes both, just stopped working at it – and believe me, it *does* need work to sustain a love.

I'm not surprised Cynthia's sex parties attracted so many guests. She was a marvellous temptress, with a wonderful sense of humour. On the sleeve of her video it says: 'Ladies, learn how you can have your own slave to do all those jobs around the home – ironing, washing, cleaning the toilet – all in return for a good smack on the bottom. And you do the smacking.'

But, seriously, you have to work at a relationship. The clever ones do it naturally and the lucky ones do it without even realizing it. If you are not in a relationship then you are not one of either of the above, but this book can change all that. And if you believe the right person just hasn't come into your life, then maybe, just maybe, you have imposed a block on your own attractions *(see case histories, Chapter 5, Elizabeth, pp.118–22).*

As well as being fortunate enough to persuade some exciting, fascinating and sophisticated people to be truthful and explicit about their own sexual experiences, my knowledge also comes through my own experience of life in the film industry as a Hollywood wife. I edited film trade papers, and specialized in interviews with film stars and the most important people in the film industry, the money men. I attended eight successive Cannes Film Festivals as a journalist and was married to an American editor who was also the author of a book entitled *Sexual Surrogate* (Henry Regnery Co., Illinois; Beaver Books, Ontario, 1976).

I had other relationships, including ones with a famous Hollywood heart-throb actor and a top British comedian. An actor called Harry Reems asked me to marry him at the Cannes Film Festival. I didn't realize at the time that he was the star of *Deep Throat*, famous for his sizeable appendage.

As a hypnotherapist, I have treated princes, ministers, judges and celebrities, also specializing in helping ordinary couples through the rough patches. All were important ingredients in my work, full of common sense psychology and peppered with information that allowed me to explore and come to terms with the most sought-after dream of the human race – a wonderful loving relationship which, of course, includes regular, lasting and satisfying sex.

However, probably the most important factor in my entire life was a six-year memory loss, which I suffered after being involved in a serious car accident. I described this fully in my previous book, *Self-Hypnosis* (Thorsons, 1994), in which I told how I decided to become a hypnotherapist myself after being cured of my amnesia by hypnosis. I was forced by an act of fate – or, indeed, literally, a road of choice – to lead a most unusual life. The experience gave me a uniqueness of information and facts, rather than theories, gained and authenticated by actually living the nightmare of a very severe memory loss. I was thus able to experience at first hand what the mind is really capable of. It was an experience which, while horrendous at the time, I now realize fitted me very well indeed for my chosen career.

Such a disabling problem gave me a whole different approach to life. For instance, I saw the value of each and every word and of using them sparingly. I discovered that, even as a cover for my amnesia, I was unable to lie. When you have a memory problem you cannot even tell white lies, because you won't remember them later! So, you tend to develop another form of manipulation, used out of necessity for survival.

I probably existed mostly using the right side of my brain, as Albert Einstein was purported to do. It was said he applied creative thinking and instinct and tended to ignore logic. By this method, you can change a situation around from what you *have* to what you *want*. You simply base your strategy on new information and forget that it may supposedly be 'impossible'.

During the years of my memory loss, I had to cope with many unusual feelings. For example, I was like a virgin every time I had sex – though whether this was a good or bad thing, I'd rather not say! I could only remember any one day at a time – and not necessarily the whole day. I could forget what had happened only seconds earlier. A national newspaper which did a story about me called it 'a 50-second memory'. The one thing that stayed constant was that I couldn't remember yesterday. In fact, I often didn't recall that yesterday had existed at all and today would have been forgotten by tomorrow. I forgot the existence of important people in my life. Friends, business associates, even my son could get lost from my mind for long periods. After a weekend trip, I would simply forget to go home. Once, I moved apartments while my boyfriend was away on a business trip. When he returned, he had no way of finding me, as I didn't leave a forwarding address. I just forgot I had a boyfriend. I was in a new place, so there was nothing to remind me of him. I never saw him again and only remembered the relationship at all a few years later when I heard a song that brought a memory back. I would just disappear out of people's lives and turn up years later when I had remembered.

My affliction gave a different edge to love-making and

relationships. My emotions were mixed – sometimes too many but mostly too few. Once I played a joke on someone which backfired on me emotionally. The man concerned was a terrible womanizer and very egotistical. A German pop singer, he was staying at the place where I was living and was outrageously flirting with me. To try and ward off his attentions, I used a trick I knew was a definite turn-off: I pretended I was in love with him and did the swooning act. Very foolish! The trouble was, I forgot it was a joke and ended up experiencing the pain of unrequited love. I actually thought I was truly in love with a person whom, if I had been in my right mind, I would have found too ridiculous for words – which shows that you can experience what you believe to be love but what in fact is mistaken identity. Years later, on reflection, I would realize that the whole thing had stemmed from a prank. Yet, on the other hand, I could genuinely be in love with someone and, as soon as I walked out of the door, forget he even existed. As you can imagine, I was very mixed up emotionally and always vulnerable for a new love. Needless to say, I had a lot of boyfriends.

I will be adding more of my experiences in the following chapters, but these exploits are included here to help you understand the often strange ways in which the mind can work. By relating them, I hope to help you look for your own solutions and, most importantly, to allow you to use the information and techniques which I learned from my own problems. 'Necessity is the mother of invention' runs the proverb. How true. I learned from my own heartbreaks, finding simple and quick techniques to prevent them happening again. Now I want to pass them on to you. The intention of this book is self-help, quick and easy to follow, so that you can create a more enjoyable existence for yourself. And why not? You deserve it.

How do people respond to the suggestion of using

self-help for greater sexual satisfaction? What complicates the situation is that people who are involved in true-love relationships are often so caught up in a euphoric 'high' that it is difficult to find any complaints – that is, they don't believe that their sex life needs, or is capable of, any improvement. The mind has totally ruled out anything negative, unless you catch one of the partners in between emotions or both in a difference of opinion. At the beginning of a relationship, there are generally no arguments – they very often come later. It is also very difficult to get the realistic view, as there are generally so many contradictions. This is highlighted in one of my case histories, Leon, in Chapter 5, who developed love into an obsession, in the end driving him to a psychiatrist. But you will find there are many links to help you understand the workings of the mind when you are in love.

In the early stages of this book, I was getting very frustrated. I would ask each couple how they rated their overall sexual and emotional height of satisfaction on a score ranging from one to ten, and I began to believe that people in a new love relationship were going to have a scale of ten out of ten forever. At least, that's what they told me and I began to believe them, knowing that it was surely possible. I did notice, however, that one partner in one of the couples I interviewed had already claimed a ten with his previous relationship. I had known him for years and remembered that he had more or less said the same thing before, until the relationship went sour. I mentioned this to him but he assured me that this new relationship was even better, more like ten-plus-plus. I wondered!

All of the couples believed that what they were experiencing was simply the best sex possible. The question is: are they capable of experiencing even better? Are they at the moment unaware there is a better? How can you know there isn't more if you've never experienced more? Thinking you already have it all is definitely left-brain logic, rather than right-brain instinct, preventing growth and keeping you tied together when things go wrong. Hypnosis, by implanting a suggestion into the mind, can do a 'spring cleaning' job, sweeping away the cobwebs so that even greater pleasure can be experienced.

I was attending an important function, so I booked an appointment to have my hair done. My hairdresser, Paul, is an extremely down-to-earth guy, good-looking, with a personality that is so friendly and charming you would feel quite comfortable telling him all your secrets. Don't they say that women tell all to their hairdresser? Well, Paul is a natural. He is surrounded by women all day, every day, and he was able to give me a comprehensive, practical view of the situation. 'We hairdressers help the medical profession,' he told me. 'Our clients tell us all their problems and so they don't need a therapist.'

I asked Paul what was the percentage of his customers at any one time in a new love relationship. He replied, 'I see this romance thing so often. The girls come in here telling me how happy they are. I see them get married. I may even be invited to the wedding. They are so full of it and really happy and I think, "Good on you," and it makes me feel good. But a year or so down the line the same person will tell me it's not working out. It happens all the time. It never seems to last. They don't necessarily leave the relationship, but boredom sets in.' I never did find out the percentage.

Boredom that both partners settle for is the most dangerous hurdle. People simply get bored with the same partners but rarely like to admit it, even to themselves. This is precisely what my doctor to the Royals had told me when I asked him what happens to the sparkle in a relationship. It's the boredom of seeing the same body every night, year after year. The men I talked to certainly agreed in this area, nodding and adding that the husband/lover never lets on to this – they just become vulnerable to another woman's flattery and even an affair. How many times do you see a husband in a TV soap opera kiss his wife on the cheek, tell her he loves her and then leave to join his mistress?

I have seen this boredom time and time again with my girlfriends, too, many of them models, beauty queens, beauty demonstrators or in other glamorous jobs. In Hollywood, you also get exactly the same sort of cycle, whether it be with secretaries, tea boys or film stars. In the beginning a relationship is wonderful and then time seems to be the enemy.

In fact, most happily married couples go through some stages of boredom, often silently and in denial, hiding it from each other and even from themselves. But the hypnotherapist is always privy to this information, as the layers of excuses are removed and the truth comes forward. This could so easily be rectified before it gets too far by couples going for hypnosis together in couples therapy. But it does take a specialist hypnotherapist to get the full benefits. Alternatively, with self-help and simple suggestions in hypnosis, you can do most of the work yourself. The therapist would then only be needed for problems that were trauma-based.

I set out to find a way to let everyone have the chance not only to experience natural ecstasy but, most of all, to be able to prolong it. I used the premise that if you can prolong something for a short length of time, then there is nothing stopping you from prolonging it for any length of time you care to choose – in fact, indefinitely.

In the mid-1980s I had been told that you could have a wonderful sex life with hypnosis and that you could actually gear yourself to fall in love, or out of love, with a popular phobia technique. At the time I needed to leave a relationship that had turned sour, more due to events rather than personality clashes. I was at a hypnotherapy convention in Los Angeles and a colleague was aware that I was stuck in the relationship, not trying to get out of it because I felt guilty at the thought of hurting my partner. It's the feeling you get when you believe you are going to break the other person's heart – which is quite egotistical really. I had been told years before how unfair it is to stay in a relationship when you know it isn't working. 'You are wasting the other person's time and stopping them from finding someone else,' I was told by a woman who had been married half a dozen times. Well, if anyone knew, I suppose she should! But remarks like this are rarely heeded and rarely help. Only after it's all over do you realize they are true, especially when you discover that your former lover's heart was only broken for a matter of months before they pulled themselves out of the emotional trauma and ego-bashing of being dumped and got on with their lives, often to the extent of finding someone else.

My colleague paid for three therapists to treat me, as he wanted to be sure I would come to my senses. I returned to the UK and shortly afterwards I was able to make the break. Hypnosis came to the rescue again.

I have had relationships since then that I have had to dispense with, but only a couple of other times have I used hypnosis to clear my mind of an unwanted love. The strange thing is that being a hypnotherapist yourself doesn't necessarily mean that you use the tools of hypnosis to enhance your own life. Some do, but most don't. This is similar to the hypnotherapist who smokes, even though their main source of income is stopping people from smoking. I decided to see if I could find out why.

Hypnotherapists will make all the excuses on earth as to why they won't use hypnosis on themselves. I believe that inwardly they are scared it won't work, which would be a blow to their confidence. This is another example of left-brain logic – and quite unfounded when they see smoker after smoker leaving their office a confirmed non-smoker.

While I was writing this book, I had 15 hypnotherapists around for a discussion on therapy. I asked how many of them had used hypnotic suggestion to help their own sex lives. Only two hands went up. One man had found that using hypnosis had not only gained him a 50 per cent increase in overall satisfaction, but he later changed his partner and married someone he was very happy with. He hadn't used it since, had never really thought to, in fact. He may have been thinking of the old American saying, 'If it ain't broke, don't fix it.' This is a colourful but true expression, but in this case maybe a hindrance. If it ain't broke, it still might work better!

WHAT IS LOVE?

No one has yet come up with any formula that explains why, or how, you fall in love, or why you are suddenly wildly attracted to another person beyond all reason. When you are in this kind of relationship, it starts out as being quite exquisite. You feel so vibrant and alive and you may even feel sorry for the people around you because they are not experiencing such wonders. You believe that anyone else who is in love cannot possibly be experiencing something as fantastic as you are. Why? Because your mind has created utopia and utopia is a place where everything is perfect.

It is later in the relationship that utopia may start to resemble hell, but only while you are experiencing the negative emotions. These can easily be brought on by petty, unreasonable jealousies or accentuated rejections. Then everything is exaggerated, every word starts to have hidden meaning and communication can become a minefield of innuendoes and misunderstandings. You need to tread carefully, as this is the dangerous time for a relationship. The thought of losing such an alive feeling, not to mention the fantastic sex, and the thought of ever finding anyone else who can make you feel so extraordinary is unthinkable. So what is going on in the mind? What happened to logic and reason?

'Mr Charming' is a client I was specifically treating for the research for this book. He agreed to allow me to use his case as an example. I will call him Adam. He has had many relationships and his last lover ditched him several months ago. He didn't expect it to happen as, although there were many problems, he believed that they would be surmounted. We found there was a pattern to his relationship behaviour. He would meet someone at a club or a function, fall head over heels for her, the girl would stay overnight and immediately afterwards would have moved in, leaving a few years later.

Adam is in his mid-thirties, good looking and the type who brings flowers on a first date. It struck me he would have to be extremely charming to get such a reaction from a girl that she would move in with him virtually straightaway. And it's not exactly a sensible beginning to a relationship. What more romantic to a girl than to be whisked off her feet and romanced by a man saying he never wants to be apart from her ever? However, it becomes less romantic when you discover that this is a pattern and the way Adam makes his mistakes, not learning, just looking and hoping, his subconscious working on a faulty or fantasy programme.

Then there was the unscrupulous charmer I knew of who used 'I want to marry you' as his introduction. He would then make long-distance calls on his mobile phone to places like Dubai and indulge in a conversation that gave the impression he was doing multi-million pound deals. The result would often be that impressionable girls would end up financing him for his next fling. The eventual separation was done so cleverly that they would never know they had been conned. He was an expert lover – but, then, that was an essential part of his stock in trade, as he worked on his bogus relationships as a business venture.

I was talking to Philip Hodson, agony aunt for *The Jimmy Young Show* on BBC Radio 2, who also writes for magazines and newspapers. He is a qualified psychotherapist and registered counsellor. He backed up my opinion that love and lust have an expiry, or sell-by, date. He gave them two years on average. According to Philip, it is far more realistic to give the lovers permission to enjoy their exciting feelings for as long as they last, rather than to base their whole lives on them. He suggests a real test of love is to wait until the conditions are not so favourable – perhaps when one partner is ill or has lost their job, or when the relationship is under pressure in some way – and see how the couple handles that situation. Philip explains: 'When the scales fall from your eyes, then you wonder what on earth you are doing with this person.' He believes that to achieve a more lasting relationship, you need to have tolerance and acceptance and actually work on the relationship, not just take it for granted.

Philip explained that because at one time people weren't expected to live long, the terms of relationships were quite short. Ten years would be the expectancy and then one or other partner would succumb to what we would now consider an early death. As public health improved, the life span of the average person increased and so relationships had to contend with these changed circumstances.

Another, more recent change has been the status of women. These days, they are not bound to men in quite the same way as in past centuries. First, more women – over 11 million – are in employment, so they have an economic life of their own.

And secondly, they are not dependent on the fact that when they have sex they are likely to have a baby. We have efficient means of contraception which are widely available and sometimes free. In 1870 you would probably not know where to get a condom and if you did, it might be very ineffective.

Philip went on:

> The only thing that is sustaining long-term relationships now is the willingness of the parties to be in them. Obviously, there are exceptions, but in some cases it's the quality of intimacy alone that keeps people going. There are all sorts of pressures these days. There's a gender battle going on between the women and men.
>
> Also, with the destabilization of the typical family in all its forms, from divorce, temptation and the disruptions of people losing their jobs to the ineffectiveness of people, people now don't have much sense of responsibility. They are copying the instability of their parents' marriage, causing a lot more separations. As a nation, we can't afford it economically, financially or from the point of view of the impact on our children. They need us to stay together, whether we need to or not.

Philip's view on intimacy is that it is not just sexual but:

> ...a feeling that somebody understands you and in the end is on your side, will put you first; a sense of partnership, of bonding. People don't talk about this when we talk about relationships. You are told from childhood: 'One day you will fall in love and get married.' Well, that's not going to take you very far unless you have learned how to *bond*, how to relate to somebody else. We don't tell kids or the world in general what makes a good relationship,

He is right. Many people in relationships are like Adam, who believed he could get away with his unacceptable behaviour and that he and his partner would manage to see it out together, thus constantly failing. In such cases, your partner will last only as long as it takes for someone else to come into their life. They are vulnerable, perhaps only staying with you out of guilt. In some cases, however, you may be unlucky enough to have this wrong relationship forever, condemned to a lifetime of dissatisfaction, frustration and boredom.

Philip added:

When people are drunk on love they should not make too many decisions, like getting married, and certainly not have children. They are like the classic drunk, not reasonable, and it is very difficult to talk to them sensibly. They believe that love conquers all, which, of course, it doesn't.

In a wonderfully descriptive phrase, Philip describes couples who are lovers-in-lust as being like 'conspirators in madness'. However, he delighted in their experiences and wished them all the best, suggesting that they enjoy it while they can. His experience as an agony aunt has led him to develop a strong scepticism. He has found the most short-lived relationships are the love-at-first-sight type. 'They are top of my list for broken hearts,' he concluded.

I also talked to Adam Cole, producer and director of the video *Love Plan*, which gives tasteful, light and informative help for lovers. He gave me his views, based on his research:

There's love and there's *need* and, of course, there is a huge gulf between them. There's only one sort of true love and that is unconditional love. However, there are all sorts of different relationships which are a reflection of themselves and their partners. I certainly know of one great love affair currently, where two people have just got together and they haven't been able to tear themselves apart from one another for a couple of years. But relationships seem to go through different stages. First, a honeymoon stage where it's very intense, the physical side is very strong and you are finding out about each other, an exploration satisfying sexual curiosity. It's all new, fresh and, in contrast to what we have had before, more stimulating. Then usually things settle down and become some type of commitment around the idea of a relationship. Then there is the power struggle, where each one is trying to get their needs met within the relationship and to establish their territory.

Classically, the men tend to control the assets and the women tend to control the bedroom activity. There's a trade-off. It's been like this since time immemorial. From prostitution on upwards, women control sex. They control sexual favours and then, broadly speaking, control their men who then, in turn, control the assets of society. Sometimes you get one person in control of everything. Once those roles get defined, everything gets set in concrete and they arrive at the dead zone. If you can try and overcome relationship problems, then sex gets a lot better. If we can start to confront our fears in intimacy, so we can feel free to be who we are. That is what intimacy is. It's acknowledging who you really are and feeling no fear about sharing with somebody else. We play roles to a huge extent in our relationships. We are eager to please. We think we have to be a certain way to be attractive and that places an enormous amount of stress on us.

To most people, sex is something that happens in

their heads. In fact, we are never in our bodies, we are in a fantasy world and there are a lot of people promoting fantasy. Fantasy is always about being somewhere else. It's not about being present and a lot of people in relationships rely on fantasy. Most people think about eating an ice cream, as opposed to really 100 per cent experiencing eating the ice cream.

Adam explained that you should take time to be in your body and experience sensations like touch, rather than just thinking about it. Peak experiences, whether they exist in classical music or climbing mountains, come to people when they are not distracted or fragmented but when all their senses are totally alert.

Adam also pointed out that sex can be used as a fix, to help sleep or relieve tension. If you have a business meeting with the bank manager the next morning, a good bout of love-making will relax you and set you up in the right frame of mind for the encounter. 'Many people see it as a performance of the macho self, which they mirror.'

DIFFERENT TYPES OF LOVE DILEMMA

Some of the different types of relationships in this next section are ones you may recognize yourself as being in, or having been in. Each one is quite different, though you may find that your relationships are a bit of each, with both positive and negative aspects.

Love and Passion at First Sight
How many people have ever actually experienced the love-at-first-sight, chemical, highly sexual and ten-on-the-emotional-Richter-scale kind of relationship? In my research

I found that only a small percentage of people seemed to have reached such a high mind-blowing sexual plateau with their partner.

To experience such ecstasy is equal only to the excitement a human being might experience in a wartime battle situation, pumping adrenalin and suffering every emotion imaginable. In a very short space of time – a week, even a day – you can go through a vast range of feelings that leave you even more stimulated and mind-blown. Remember, adrenalin is addictive. Laughter, crying, jealousy, hate, undying love can all be experienced almost simultaneously and repeated in a seemingly endless spiral of events. Usually, this treadmill of emotions lasts as long as the relationship itself. The down side is that very often other things go to pot, because the whirlwind love affair leaves very little time to concentrate on your profession or business affairs. Such powerful emotions may be beautiful while they last but they can also create unreasonable behaviour, sometimes resulting in despair and even tragedy.

To be involved in the sort of sexual fixation which is usually mistaken for ultimate love can be very dangerous and can lead to crime and/or illness when your lover leaves. In fact in France the special offence of a 'crime of passion' is recognized. It is counted as a crime with special mitigating circumstances and punishments can be very lenient, even for murder. The reasoning is that the mind of the offender is considered unbalanced at the time of the crime.

Still, few people seem to know of the existence of such overwhelming feelings. I have spoken to many eminent people and experts in relationships who have never experienced them at all. A sizeable percentage of the population believes such highs and lows are peculiar to romantic novels and movies like *Gone with the Wind* (which portrays such feelings excellently). If you are one of these people, you are very wrong. I can assure you that the experiences detailed in so many works of fiction can happen in reality and are as old as time. They may sound unrealistic to the average person but they can happen to anyone if the right buttons have been pressed – chemically, that is.

Knowing that level of pleasure exists is only half the story. What is more exciting is that now certain negative emotions can be eliminated and replaced with positive ones, allowing you to take out the destructive feelings, such as jealousies and other illogical hurts. These negative emotions only plunge the relationship into jeopardy. Banish them and you leave in their place that wonderful feeling of ecstasy, naturally produced and beautifully balanced, simply by changing the strategy of the subconscious.

So, whether you are in a highly emotionally charged relationship or a more laid-back one, the rules are the same. You can adjust and balance out emotions to your comfort and satisfaction. It is important to form a certain balance, so that you can experience all forms of sexual excitement with an equilibrium that is beneficial, rather than destructive.

If you have experienced the high tension kind of relationship, then you can draw from the experience and rekindle the sexual highs with another partner, even if the signs of such sexual joy are not yet apparent. That's the beauty and power of self-hypnosis. You can have a wonderful sex life with any partner you chose, with a little help from hypnosis. But only, of course, if your subconscious is assured it would be in your ultimate interests.

Let me explain this sort of relationship which is at the top of the sexual emotions scale. In itself, the relationship becomes a sexual addiction which is reserved for that special partner and you know with absolute certainty that they feel the same chemistry – no other person has a look in with either of you. However rich or famous, attractive or exciting any other person you come into contact with during this extraordinary mind-blowing relationship, they wouldn't stand a chance. They would be an intruder. However, even with this knowledge you still can become jealous with a frightening intensity.

The partner who has had such an impact on your whole life does not have to be particularly attractive, but to you they are wonderful. You become so tuned in to them that your whole existence is balanced on the question: 'How long will it be before I see them?' Time seems to stretch into infinity and a day apart from your lover becomes a lifetime.

In fact, your life is on hold when they are not with you. No longer can you enjoy your favourite hobbies or pastimes in the carefree way you once did. Your job, even if it was previously completely fulfilling, now takes a back seat to this constant sexual stirring. In company, only to touch your lover's skin for reassurance helps sustain you until you can retire to spend hours performing every sexual pleasure possible.

You call it love – what else could it be?! You suddenly understand what the saying 'seeing your lover through rose-coloured spectacles' means. They can say or do no wrong in your eyes. Even if smoking is normally a turn-off to you, seeing them doing it looks good. However, this applies only to your lover and not to others. You are ignoring the contradiction and conflict in your mind, defying its illogicality. This leaves no room for unconditional love because all your buttons have been pressed and your emotions are in complete turmoil, scrambled. Logic meantime goes out the window, rarely to return.

If you recognize these symptoms, then you are more than likely thankful to be out of this acute turmoil of a relationship that usually finishes in tears, hurt and anger. If you are in the middle of one, then you need some tips to help you sustain or survive it.

A major problem that can make things even worse – or may be the core of it – is that without realizing it you may not be compatible with the person you desire so much, the person you are so chemically tuned in with. If, on the other hand, you are one of the rare lucky ones and you are extremely compatible as well – which is probably as chancy as winning the jackpot prize in the lottery – then keep this book handy in case by some quirk of fate in the future your happiness is taken away, or you simply want to keep it generating but more comfortably.

If you've loved and lost, by your own choice or your partner's, I will give you hints on how to reach that sexual high with someone else, even though it may seem at the moment impossible. The impossible is always possible with hypnosis. Once your body has experienced such sensations, by using mind games via hypnosis the memory can be re-established at will with even the most unlikely partner.

As already mentioned, you can also fall in or out of love with the use of hypnosis techniques. I'm sure Shakespeare knew the power of hypnosis when he wrote some of his plays. There is a perfect example in *A Midsummer Night's Dream* in the scene in which a love potion is administered to the Fairy Queen Titania, causing her to fall in love with the first person she sees when she awakes. This turns out to be Bottom, who has been given the head of an ass by Oberon, the Fairy King. Doesn't that remind you of stage hypnosis, in which willing subjects do whatever the hypnotist tells them to, however outrageous? Incidentally, there is no need to use preconditioned subjects to act out the antics on stage. It is very basic hypnosis and as long as the subject is willing to play – as that's precisely what they are doing – then you can easily make someone believe you are their favourite sex symbol. Many an unscrupulous stage hypnotist has used this ploy to indulge in a long kiss and cuddle on the stage with a beautiful girl. The girl isn't very happy afterwards, realizing she has kissed a frog!

Hypnosis is very powerful. In the USA stage hypnotists can bring females on stage to orgasm. I can assure you that it is very possible, which proves you can create a climax even without imagination. Simply a quick hypnotic suggestion that you will experience a climax is enough. The subconscious just brings that memory forward and activates the body. It will happen and it does. The subject can always come out of hypnosis, but generally they don't, possibly because of a mixture of curiosity and not believing it has a chance of working. When it does, they are intrigued that they have been able to command on thought such an experience. In fact, they just enjoy the experience without any inhibitions. That's in general, of course. I am not giving my views or opinions on this rather strange phenomenon, just reporting what I have experienced at first hand. You can probably understand from this how a molested child or rape victim can have sexual excitement attached to fear and/or pain. Later, however, confusing and warped sexual preferences can be created instead of warm and wonderful emotions, spoiling what could have been a healthy and wonderful sex life.

If you are a sceptic and think that this is all just stuff in story-books, then you should either open your mind and be prepared to activate an experience that is mind-blowing or bury your head in the sand. It is your choice.

Unconditional Love

This is so often misinterpreted. It becomes a 'love dilemma' if you believe it simply means that you put the other person's happiness before yours and mean it, even if you have to remove yourself from the relationship altogether, making a complete sacrifice for their happiness and well-being. You then sit on the sidelines, hoping that they will want you back, which is quite possible, but you are so in love that you will accept whatever they want, even if it means that they may meet someone else. Jealousy is around and can be very focused, but not so intense that you can't handle it. Such a relationship can be beautiful, romantic and wonderful, but you may suffer a great deal of despair as you go through the treadmill of emotions. You also place a guilt trip on your partner which does not leave room for your letting go and finding someone else. It might be wise to consider the fact that if the relationship has broken up before, it was probably wrong anyway. And unless you both change dramatically, then it's just a matter of time before it goes wrong again. You are really trying to mend something which may not be simply damaged but permanently broken.

The Perfect Match

I have done therapy with couples who give the impression that they are the perfect match. To all their friends, they have a perfect life together. But it isn't all it seems. I am not saying that there aren't people who have actually managed to get it right, who have a wonderful and balanced compatibility that leaves room for each of their personalities to grow separately, as well as growing closer together – but there aren't many. Often couples love each other yet live through conflict all of their lives in a sort of love-hate relationship. If you take away the bickering and the hurt, there's little time for pleasure. The negativity is taking its toll in time and energy. I have been in this type of relationship and when it ends it's quite a relief.

Caring Behaviour

I spoke to Professor Lucas, Keeper of the Herbarium at the world-famous Kew Gardens, who was adviser to David Attenborough's wonderful book *The Living Plants*.

I wanted to see if I could learn something from plant life and whether there really are any parallels with human behaviour. After all, isn't Prince Charles always telling us we should love our plants and nurture them by talking to them? But Professor Lucas is very sceptical of this theory. He explained that in his experience the person looking after the plants does not have to have any love or compassion for them. As long as that person knows what they need and gives it to them, catering for their needs in the form of water, food and correct conditions, they respond and grow just as healthily as they would if someone really loved and nurtured them.

It reminded me of some people I know. They presume they are loved because their partner always cares for them. But it doesn't mean they are *unconditionally loved* and they get a terrible shock when the partner leaves them and moves on. To be able to keep that love and sparkle alive and not to take for granted that we will be loved forever without any effort, we have to work at it. Love needs to be nurtured and, like plants, it needs feeding and sometimes it needs vitamins to keep it healthy.

REPROGRAMMING YOURSELF

Human beings are programmed to discover and formulate strategies to get what they want. It's a natural instinct from birth. A baby may find that it gets its own way by being calm and quiet, while another baby finds it doesn't get its own way quite so easily and so tries other strategies, like screaming and throwing tantrums. The early pattern usually stays and the first baby grows up to be a pleasant adult, niceness and kindness being its key to getting what it wants, while the other child grows up to be not so pleasant and even downright obnoxious, still screaming at others for what it wants for itself.

Wouldn't it be smart to mentally reprocess the unpleasantness in yourself to act pleasantly, programming yourself in such a way that you do it without thinking, so that you are more likely to give back into life instead of just taking?

You can also preprogramme your body to encourage an encounter of a magnificent kind. You don't have to be beautiful, attractive or confident even, but you must wish, and expect, it to happen. This programmes your subconscious to prepare and send out signals that you and the people around you are aware of. It happens at a deep level, rather like the whistle the dog can hear but human beings can't.

Being a one-time journalist, I usually subscribe to the statement: 'Believe nothing that you read and only half of what you see.' The remark became very appropriate when I recently met the idol of my teenage years, pop singer Emile Ford. I was delighted to meet him at a celebrity party and was able to talk to him about my teenage thrills from his live performances in the 1960s. I certainly wasn't prepared for what he told me, as he was explaining how he was able to perform so sincerely. The sexuality oozing from the stage as he knelt on one knee to sing his love ballads was actually *focused sincerity*. He couldn't see much of the audience in the darkened theatre, so he imagined he was singing to children, a group he was used to performing for. As children have a short attention span, he needed to 'act' his songs out and he did this with sincerity rather than a childish strutting around the stage – children are, after all, little adults. So he used focused attention to keep the fans mesmerized. All that sex was in the imagination of the audience. The love in his songs was not about sex, but beauty. It was his audience that presumed it was sexuality oozing from him, when in fact it was pure emotion, focused and sincere.

I remember when I was five years old my mother told me that you cannot look someone straight in the eye and lie. I'm afraid I found out that she was wrong! You *could* look someone in the eye and tell the most gigantic fibs. I did not become an inveterate liar, but I did become a very good salesperson. I would look very sincere and caring, while more than likely I would be thinking about what shopping I needed to do or where my next call would be. A good salesperson usually becomes a master of deception, especially if working on commission only.

Doesn't this remind you of the clever seducer who swears undying love on the first date, perhaps with a little alcohol helping the look of sincerity, only for the unfortunate victim to find out too late that it was all just a spiel to get them into bed? The patter rarely varies – indeed, word for word it is often identical – with each potential victim vulnerable and ripe for feeling loved or lovable.

Some people fall for the wrong partners constantly. The pattern never changes. It is a learned programme that has been activated through an experience way back in past. All that the unfortunate person realizes is that they are in another familiar mess, constantly getting involved with the wrong people and inviting calamity and tears for the future – programmed for disaster, in fact. Wouldn't it be wonderful to change the programme?

You will find that in this book there are carefully selected hypnotic suggestion scripts that you can mix and match so that you can create a suggestion that is just right for you. The power of suggestion is amazing and can be used for your benefit over and over again, clearing problems as they become focused. To use my own example, whilst I spend much of my life helping others, I find I need to have regular therapy myself, mainly because my life is quite complicated as I am constantly surrounded by the unusual. I call it 'spring cleaning the mind'. You can do it too. Your life is in your hands.

TWO

Hypnosis is a mind massage
in which the words are used to stroke the mind

This chapter has been designed as a simple guide on how to hypnotize yourself. Or if you wish, you can ask your lover or a trusted friend to help. Working together can be fun, allowing you to create your own custom-designed therapy. However it is not necessary to work with someone else. You might prefer to do it privately – it depends on you. The next two chapters will help you in whichever way you choose. I have listed the instructions and tools for you to acquire excellent hypnosis, a type of DIY self-help therapy to allow your mind to be persuaded to change certain unwanted attitudes or old programmes, so you can enjoy a healthier sex life. By 'healthier', I mean mentally creating a clear road to satisfaction.

The purpose of going into a trance is to enable the inner mind to accept instructions that will encourage greater inner stability in sexual involvements, while clearing out old unwanted fears and doubts – mental cobwebs, if you like. It's a little like getting rid of the cobwebs in a room, the ones you hadn't noticed behind the couch because they had been hidden from view, perhaps for years.

A little reprogramming can do a clean-up job on negativity, giving you control of your own mind. Think of your mind as being like a computer and imagine you have just bought some new software. You hire a computer expert to show you what to do. As he points to the keys you need to press, you don't get nervous and think he is some kind of god because he can work something that you can't. He has had to learn, like you, and this is what this book is about – teaching you to use your head.

Hypnosis is probably one of the most misunderstood therapies. People still cling to old misguided beliefs. Even some hypnotherapists are, regrettably, unwilling to change their outdated views, which they probably picked up from old-fashioned books or simply misunderstood in the first place. For every good book on the subject, there are many bad ones.

To give an example of the kind of misinformation that exists, I have had many clients who say they have been told they can't be hypnotized. This is a very common misconception. Usually, it occurs because they are not a visual person; they can't actually see things in their imagination but just 'know' what something looks like. When the hypnotherapist tells them to picture something or see it in hypnosis – without establishing if the person is visual or not before the hypnosis – the subject worries that because they can't actually picture something they are not in hypnosis. In fact, it's just a lack of communication between a visual hypnotherapist and non-visual client. It never happens the other way around. A non-visual person always knows exactly how a visual person will react. Before embarking on any treatment, I always conduct a simple test to find out whether the client is visual or not.

There are two very important facts that you should know...

First, everyone – everyone, that is, who is conscious and not suffering from brain damage – can be hypnotized.

Anyone who thinks otherwise is ignorant of the basics of hypnosis and doesn't understand it. Every time you go into a daydream you are, in fact, in hypnosis. And, since everybody daydreams dozens of times in a normal day, then it stands to reason you are capable of being hypnotized.

It was once believed that people who are insane couldn't be hypnotized. The problem here is not getting them into hypnosis, but getting them out of their own little world into reality. It was also believed that you couldn't hypnotize someone if you didn't speak their language. That is also a fallacy. There are now new techniques to get over this problem. I have seen it done, both in America and by a Russian scientist/hypnotherapist.

Another misconception, which has led to much unreasonable fear of hypnosis, is that you can be made to do something against your will when you are hypnotized. I researched this very thoroughly, so I could answer without fear of being misguided myself.

I arranged to interview Alan Sheflin in his home in San Francisco. He is considered one of the US's foremost experts in hypnotherapy, with a BA in psychology, a Masters in Law and an LLM and MA in counselling psychology. He is a celebrated lecturer and author, winning the prestigious Guttmacher award from the American Psychiatry Association for the finest publication on forensic psychology. His views are highly regarded by the medical profession and the layman alike. One of his books on mind manipulation and brainwashing techniques was used virtually as a manual by the CIA and other intelligence agencies.

I asked Sheflin to confirm my own view – which he did – that, as long as you are made aware of it, you can say 'No' in hypnosis; you cannot be made to do things you wouldn't normally do. If a person is made to do something against their will, he told me, then that is brainwashing and hypnosis is only a small part of the equation. Drugs, and sometimes the inflicting of pain, play a far more relevant part in brain-washing techniques than hypnosis.

Let me give you an example of what I mean. If it were possible to brainwash someone in hypnosis, I could probably become very rich very quickly indeed! How? I would simply be able to instruct clients that when they came out of hypno-sis they would go to the bank, take out all their money and give it to me. Then, I would add to that an instruction for them to forget the previous instruction, just as the stage hypnotist does with his willing volunteers.

The information or induction given to the subject before the actual hypnosis is very important, so it would be beneficial for you to read this book thoroughly before you actually commence your home therapy. Even the case histories in Chapter 5 are designed to give you more knowledge of the inner workings of the mind, expanding your own thoughts and proving how different the inner mind's logic is in comparison with the conscious.

Even if you already know quite a lot about hypnosis, it is always an advantage to see a different point of view. That is what each technique is, a different approach to get to the cause of the problem.

You may not have a problem as such in your sexual rela-tionship, but just want to experience the hypnotic techniques to enhance an already exciting sexual relationship. Even so, these studies will allow you to look more closely at what you may have previously taken for granted, giving you the ammunition to adjust and fine tune your feelings and emotions. Think of it, as already suggested, as a 'spring cleaning of the mind'.

HYPNOSIS SUCCESS RATES

In hypnotherapy, some techniques are better than others. To find out which are the best to use is not easy, because every hypnotherapist believes that their methods are certainly the best. You really need to know the number of sessions that it takes and balance it against a definite success rate. This is difficult because many hypnotherapists presume their clients are *fixed* – i.e., cured – without checking a few months after the therapy. It's no use having one session that will either be a short fix or not work at all. A permanent change is what we are after.

This book teaches suggestion hypnosis and you need a guideline for percentage of success. One of the largest ever scientific comparisons of the use of hypnosis was reported in the *New Scientist* in October 1992 in an extensive research project on stopping smoking. It is easy to check a smoker's behavioural change – they either smoke or they don't. Out of 72,000 people, in more than 600 studies, it was found that hypnosis was the most successful prevention on the market, even with tapes with not very good suggestions. It worked better than any other strategy – even nicotine patches.

The most important information that came out of this study was that it gave a success rate for suggestion hypnosis. This was proven to have, at worst, a 30 per cent success rate. Every other smoking 'cure' on the market is well below this. The chairman of the British Society of Medical and Dental Hypnosis, Christopher Pattinson, said this figure could double if good suggestion were used. So, therefore, you can expect that if you follow the instructions in this book you have a chance of between 30 and 60 per cent success rate for change, which is pretty good. It's strange these data often seem to have been forgotten when people say that there is no scientific research that establishes a success rate for hypnosis. They haven't obviously done their homework. Check out the national Quit Smoking line and ask for the hynotherapy success rate!

Going to a specialist in advanced hypnotherapy will give you an even better percentage of success – but you might as well try self-hypnosis first and save yourself some expense. Then, if you are not satisfied, at least you will have cut down the number of therapy sessions needed by having already done much of the work.

Most of my own problems have been mastered by sugges-tion hypnosis alone. They included fear of dragonflies, fear of noises in the night, wanting to stop drinking, giving up sugar and milk in my coffee and tea, falling out of love, clearing hurt, trebling my reading speed, writing my books and much, much more. Even hypnotherapists can have a string of problems!

HOW DOES HYPNOSIS WORK?

So, how does suggestion hypnosis work? It is important to know when the circumstances are more favourable for the suggestions to be acceptable.

Suggestions are more likely to be accepted when you are relaxed than when you are anxious. It is of little value wait-ing for a telephone call or someone to arrive when you put yourself into hypnosis, as you will not be able to relax prop-erly. So help yourself by putting aside some uninterrupted time, perhaps after your main meal in the evening or just before you start the day, but certainly not when you are late or if it may hold you up, because you will not be in the right frame of mind.

Forgive me imposing just a little technical information

upon you, but a little knowledge about the mind can help you understand why you should be relaxed. During a 24-hour period, your brain experiences four basic wave patterns: beta, alpha, theta and delta. The beta wave is the state you are in when you are awake and getting on with your daily life. The alpha wave occurs just before you go to sleep and as you awake from sleep. The theta state follows the alpha state, when you are very drowsy. When you actually fall asleep you are experiencing delta waves. So hypnosis occurs when you are in either alpha or theta, but never in delta. Quite simply, while you are asleep you are not in hypnosis. It's a fallacy believed by many that when you are in hypnosis you are asleep or unconscious – that's nonsense. When you are in a daydream you are experiencing hypnosis, when your brain waves have slowed down enough through relaxation to be in either alpha or theta.

The concept of depth or degrees of depth has little to do with the effectiveness of hypnosis. You are either in hypnosis or you are not. It's like pregnancy – you cannot be a little bit pregnant; you either are or you are not. You can never be a little bit in hypnosis either. So don't make the mistake of saying that the hypnosis didn't work because you weren't in deep enough. However, having said that, there is no denying that for most people it is a wonderful feeling to be in deep relaxation.

During the alpha state, your mind and body are completely relaxed and the supply of oxygen to your brain is increased with deep breathing. The brain waves that can be measured on an electroencephalogram (EEG) drop from 13 to 8 cycles per second. In this state your mind is ready to accept suggestions. Through brain-wave training, that is, training in hypnosis, you can increase your creative abilities and instruct your mind to sustain a good relationship. It will become very creative and form new strategies to cater for your new behaviour. In Russia, schools use hypnosis to teach children difficult language dialects and the most effective learning is produced in this state.

It is important to relax and use deep breathing, which has a very soothing effect on the body. It helps you to relax naturally, as the breathing concentration in itself stills the mind. In the progressive relaxation shown on pp.43–5, the instructions will be to relax the voluntary skeletal muscles, toes, calves, thighs, etc. As you do the relaxation exercises, blood lactate, a substance produced by the metabolic activity of skeletal muscles, is reduced and muscle tension decreases. Anxiety is caused by skeletal muscle contraction, but relaxation reverses this state. During this time, your body cells need less oxygen, your metabolism slows down and deep relaxation is the result.

Visualization is the language of the subconscious part of the mind, or the inner mind. Creating a mental picture of some carefree place will contribute to your relaxation. This is the basis of painless surgery or dental work – causing the mind to be occupied and focused on a favourite scene. There is a vast difference between consciously suggesting to yourself that you do something and directing yourself in a focused awareness (hypnosis). When your mind is relaxed enough, it is ready to accept suggestions unconditionally, but it will only accept suggestions that are not harmful to you or against your principles.

HOW TO HYPNOTIZE YOURSELF

To hypnotize yourself you need to record your voice on a tape recorder, so that you can play it back when you are relaxed. You can then chose either to play this privately or invite your lover to join you, reading your chosen scripts below or designing your own as described in the next chapter.

It doesn't make any difference whether you use the first person (I) or third person (you) when you are reading the script onto tape for yourself or your partner. It's really a matter of preference.

How You and your Lover Can Enjoy Hypnosis Together

This is a wonderful option for lovers, as it gives you the chance to pamper each other by using hypnosis as you would a wonderfully relaxing massage. In fact, hypnosis can be likened to a mind massage, the words stroking your inner mind and lulling you into a beautiful, deep relaxation.

To treat yourself to a session of hypnosis is absolutely wonderful before love-making. Of course, it is not essential to use hypnosis each and every time you make love, but it is much better if you can repeat the process often. Normally, it takes about three weeks to form the habit of doing it regularly.

First, select one of the scripts, either a general one for you both or individual ones. You can read the prepared script directly to your lover, then ask them to return the favour and read your chosen script to you. Alternatively, play your specially made recording for both of you to listen to. For the best effect, make sure you are comfortable and warm and in a room that you specially like.

By reading the scripts to each other, instead of relying on a tape, you are more in control or 'pacing' the hypnotic suggestion. This way you can guide your voice level and the speed at which you are talking to link in with your partner's breathing. Your voice should be slow and monotonous, slowing down even more when you count down into deeper relaxation. It is important to take this seriously and not to giggle or make a joke of it.

You can easily read the scripts to your lover, as you will have instructed them to close their eyes and listen and keep their eyes closed until you direct them to open them again at the end of the script. As long as you read well, without stuttering, and develop a monotonous tone while highlighting certain important words, then you will be successful.

It would be wise to familiarize yourself with the script beforehand and rehearsing it a few times would be useful, even taping it to make sure you can listen critically. Take the same trouble as you would if you had been asked to read out a passage in front of an audience. If you have put sufficient effort and thought into it beforehand, then there is no reason why you shouldn't achieve as good a trance as any professional hypnotherapist. There are no other tricks to it. The smoother your voice is and the more you glide it along the words, the better. I mentioned a monotonous tone, but you don't have to speak too slowly. Just use your common sense. When you are practising, either with or without a tape recorder, ask yourself if this would be relaxing to you if someone else were reading the script. If the answer is 'Yes', then the tape has been done correctly.

The four-step programme below gives you the correct procedure for wonderful hypnosis. So, whether you record your voice reading the scripts and play them back as you relax, or have a script read to you by your partner, you can create excellent trance.

The following are the four steps to trance:

1 The induction
2 A deepener
3 The main suggestion
4 Counting out of hypnosis

THE INDUCTION

The induction is the set of words that you use to induce a trance in preparation for the hypnotic suggestion. There are three ways to induce trance. The first two would be used by a professional hypnotherapist and the third, a slower, progressive technique, is the one I will be focusing on here. Since the first two types of induction have little relevance to this book, I will explain them only briefly, purely so that you have a fuller picture of the different types of induction that are possible.

The Instant Method

This is used primarily in the USA and is very dynamic and spectacular. Since stage hypnosis has become so popular, I find it very useful myself for demonstrations. In the UK the instant induction is used mainly by stage hypnotherapists who have very little time to spend on the induction. A sudden and unexpected physical action by the hypnotist, such as seizing the back of the subject's head and pulling it onto their shoulder, usually accompanied by a confusing order, literally shocks the mind into instant trance. Then the subject is prepared for suggestions.

Shock, by itself, is usually caused by crisis, a trauma for example. Witnessing an accident is often enough to induce a trance. When a person is badly injured and in shock, they are actually in a trance. Medics at an accident scene may not realize it, but when tending a victim they may unwittingly use a hypnotic suggestion. They can give positive suggestions to prevent the victim going into a further state of shock, which can lead to death. Remarks like 'Help is on its way' or similarly positive reassurances can help save the victim's life.

On the other hand, a careless negative remark by a passer-by – for example, 'He's got no face left!' – could be so damaging that the victim's body could go into such a state of shock that they die before they reach the hospital. It has been found that a large percentage of fatalities at the scene of an accident could have been prevented by stopping the person from going into shock.

Suggestions in shock are so powerful that you can produce changes in the physical condition directing the flow of blood. Suppose a person has a bad wound and there is dirt and grit clogging it up in the first stages of shock. Shock is responsible for preventing the flow of blood immediately after an accident. You may have probably experienced this yourself when accidentally injuring yourself, suffering a big gash that doesn't bleed immediately. You can use the trance state to get the system going and a suggestion from a responsible, believable person, for example a medic or nurse, that the flow of blood commences to clean out the wound and stops when this has been accomplished will work fine. The person in shock is not able to make the suggestion themselves because in shock thought processing has broken down. But the suggestions will be accepted, if, indeed, they are acceptable to the subconscious. This technique has been medically proven and used by medics at accident scenes in the USA for many years. It surely gives a wonderful insight into the power of suggestion hypnosis.

It follows, then, that hypnosis can be used to instruct a bodily function such as climaxing in sexual intercourse. This would be a great boon for a man who suffers with premature ejaculation or a woman who cannot climax until the man has finished. Therefore, this technique could have great possibilities for treating sexual dysfunction.

The Rapid Induction

This can be a very useful technique and is still very quick to take effect. Its basis is to confuse the mind so that it just closes down. Three easy-sounding instructions that are really complicated and cause confusion will generally do the trick. Used with confidence by an experienced hypnotherapist, this induction gives a very smooth, professional performance.

Unfortunately, you need someone to do this for you, so for self-help I will focus on the progressive induction. This simple, quick method ensures good hypnosis and all you need is a script that is read aloud.

The Progressive Induction

This is the simplest induction to use and is ideal for self-hypnosis. The words guide the subject into hypnosis. Therefore it can be self-induced or achieved via cassette tapes and you don't have to have another person present to guide you into hypnosis. You can simply listen to a pre-recording, either bought or prepared by yourself. However, it is far more effective – and more fun, too! – if you can enlist the aid of your partner.

This induction is literally an exercise in relaxation, with many different words to entice a reaction and participation. For example, the words may suggest: 'Tighten your calf muscles.' The instruction occupies the conscious while relaxing the mind, allowing the suggestion to be accepted. As the instructions become monotonous, the mind relaxes even more. It is actually *boring* the person into hypnosis. It is better to keep the words varied to help keep the attention, although certain words can be repeated regularly, for example, 'down', 'know' or 'relaxing'.

As already mentioned, the progressive relaxation technique

gradually slows down the metabolism of the subject and so, however stressed or tense they may be at the beginning, it eventually ensures a relaxation that is adequate enough to be followed by the appropriate suggestion. As long as the problem isn't trauma based and the suggestion is in the subject's interest, the new programme will then be accepted. You can always prevent yourself going into hypnosis if you are unhappy about it by refusing to relax, otherwise there is no reason why the suggestion shouldn't work.

Time spent worrying about whether you are achieving hypnosis or not is just wasted. Just let your mind drift with the words and expect it to happen. Remember, there is no feeling in hypnosis and you don't need full concentration. Just listen and relax. As soon as you begin to use your imagination you are in a form of trance, which is hypnosis.

Inductions

The following are a selection of inductions that can be used to induce hypnosis. They have been selected to suit different personalities.

Just read your chosen script into a tape recorder, either to play back to yourself or together with your lover. In order to get the full benefit, make sure you will not be disturbed. Do remember to switch your mobile phone off, if you have one, and put the ordinary telephone on silence or the answering machine. Alternately, you can ask your lover to read the script to you, lulling you into hypnosis. A third possibility is to ask a trusted third party to read it to you both.

It is better if you can listen twice a week for three weeks, as this will develop a habit and get you accustomed to the idea of instilling a new programme in your mind. Whichever method you choose, do make sure that you are feeling relaxed and comfortable and that there will be no interruptions.

Your chosen inductions can be long or short, flowery or precise and to the point. Each person will have their own idea of what is more suitable for their own personality. If you are not sure which one to chose, the first script listed below is the safest for ensuring a good hypnotic trance.

When choosing a script, check to discover whether you and/or your lover are visual. The visual partner will find they prefer a more descriptive script, whereas the non-visual lover may find this quite tedious. It is best to do a test here to check how you use your imagination.

Close your eyes and think of a chair, any chair. See what colour it is, check what it is made of, then open your eyes. Ask yourself how you visualized the chair, whether you actually saw it as in a picture or whether you just 'knew' what it looked like. Any time you are asked to picture or imagine something in hypnosis, do it in the same way as you did the chair.

I am one of those people who are not visual and have to struggle along with not 'seeing' but 'knowing' how something I am trying to imagine looks – but it still works. As already mentioned, we non-visual people are the ones who were told we couldn't be hypnotized, probably because when we were asked if we could see a picture and we would say we couldn't, the therapist thought we were being awkward. Considering that in any group of people in the Western world there are normally two thirds who are visual against one third who are not, the chances were that the therapist was visual and just didn't understand how we did it.

Now for the actual induction script, which will lead you into hypnosis...

Progressive Relaxation Induction Script

'*I want you to imagine that you're checking your body to ensure you become totally relaxed ... as your muscles relax ... just let your mind relax also ... begin with your feet ... feel your toes ... stretch them ... feel the texture of what your feet are resting on ... begin to tighten your calves ... now relax them ... let that relaxation spread past your ankles ... up your calves to the back of your knees ... feel those muscles easing ... resting comfortably ... now your thighs ... pull them tight ... be aware of those long muscles tensing ... now relax those muscles ... feel them lengthening and resting ... feel your legs sinking even deeper into the comfortable surface you are relaxing on ... now your stomach muscles ... pull them together gently ... now let them expand and relax comfortably.*

Your shoulders and back muscles ... flex your shoulders ... feel those muscles pull across your back ... now let your shoulders slouch as you relax the muscles ... and notice how your spine sinks deeper into your resting-place... as you relax even more deeply ... notice how easy and regular your breathing has become ... now your fingertips ... and fingers ... clench them ... feel that tension ... now relax them ... and allow the relaxation to spread up your arms to your neck ... make sure your neck is comfortable, with your head in an easy position ... tighten up your neck muscles ... now let them loosen up ... as the muscles relax ... allow your neck to shrink into a comfortable position ... your face muscles are flat and stretch comfortably across your face ... squeeze up your face ... and feel the tension ... now relax those muscles and feel them lengthening ... and softening ... relaxing ... more than ever before.

Now you can feel the air temperature against your skin ... it feels smooth and comfortable ... now you can allow the relaxation to spread to your scalp ... knowing that you are relaxed throughout your body ... from the top of your head ... to the tips of your toes.

Your body is now loose ... and limp ... and heavy ... and relaxed ... notice how your body is sinking deeper into relaxation ... as your breathing becomes more regular and easy ... in a moment I will count slowly from one ... to ten ... and with each number you will drift ... deeper ... and deeper ... into peaceful relaxation ... one ... two ... three ... four ... five ... six ... seven ... eight ... nine ... ten [count slowly and deliberately].

You are now feeling so deeply relaxed ... you find it easy to focus your attention ... and imagine things very clearly ... and I want you to imagine that you are standing on a balcony ... which has steps leading down to a beautiful garden ... as you look into the garden ... you see that it is surrounded by lovely trees ... ensuring the garden is private ... secluded ... and peaceful ... there are flower beds ... set in the lawn ... and further along is a waterfall ... flowing into a stream ... listen to the sound of the water ... as you look around ... you see the trees ... and you hear a faint sound of a bird in the distance ... adding to the feeling of deep ... relaxation ... throughout your entire being.

If you look more closely you will see that there are five steps leading down to the garden ... and then a small path ... which leads to the waterfall ... in a moment we will walk down the steps ... and with each step you go deeper ... and deeper into relaxation ... so let's begin ... watch your foot as you place it on to the first step ... and as you do this you feel yourself going deeper into relaxation ... down on to the second step ... and as you feel your foot firmly placed on the step ... you feel a wonderful relief ... as you drift even deeper into relaxation ... down on to the third step ... feeling wonderfully free and ... so ... so ... relaxed ... as your foot reaches for the fourth step ... another wave of relaxation drifts through your whole body ... down on to the fifth step now ... and feeling even more deeply relaxed than ever before.

Now you are standing on the lawn ... you see a little way ahead ... is a waterfall ... and at the side of it ... is a garden bench ... notice the colour of the bench ... what it is made of ... in a moment I would like you to walk over to the bench ... and sit down on it ... when you sit down you will be surprised at how comfortable it is ... and then you will be even more relaxed than you are now.

So let's begin to walk over ... now sit down on the bench ... and as you sit down on the bench ... take a deep breath ... and as you breathe out ... you feel a wave of relaxation go through your body ... relaxing every muscle and nerve ... as you breathe in ... you breathe in positive thoughts ... and as you breathe out ... you breathe out negative thoughts ... leaving room for more positive thoughts.'

Counting Out of Hypnosis

At the end of your induction and suggestion, and of any other work that you will be doing, when it is time to come out of hypnosis you can just add the following words:

'In a moment I will count from ten down to one, and at the count of one your eyes will open.'

An Alternative Progression Induction (Beach Fantasy)

'Picture yourself on a beautiful ... serene ... beach ... by the ocean ... the sky is clear and blue overhead ... some birds are floating gently on the breeze ... the rhythmic sounds of the waves breaking on the shore creates a wonderful wave of relaxation that seems to wash over you ... the temperature is just perfect for you ... as your toes play gently in the soft sand.

As you look around ... you notice that along the beach in the distance is a large rock ... you want to see the rock closer ... you walk gracefully and effortlessly towards the rock ... the sun is shining gently on your back ... there is a gentle breeze refreshing you ... every now and then an extra surge from the sea rushes up the beach and runs over your feet ... the sea is just the right temperature for you to enjoy its tingling feel.

As you approach the rock you start to feel an even more pleasant relaxation ... it flows over you ... every step you take towards the rock makes you feel even more relaxed than you were before ... finally, you reach the rock ... and you notice a few steps that lead to the top ... you decide to climb them ... as you take each step a question that you have been holding onto in your mind becomes clearer and clearer ... when you reach the top of the rock everything becomes even more beautiful than before ... and as you stand there absorbing the beauties and wonders of nature ... a lovely melody seems to come out of the rock itself ... floating in the breeze ... the very melody gives you an answer ... an answer to the question that was earlier on your mind.

As you are so relaxed ... it is easy for you to imagine

a wonderful romantic and loving relationship ... this is a special picture ... you can create the scene ... direct your own romantic movie ... staring yourself ... and your partner ... you find that you can direct yourself easily ... everything becomes clear to you ... you see earlier mistakes ... and you notice how easily they can be rectified with a change of thought and body language ... you direct yourself with confidence and clarity ... and this scene stays with you ... when you return to full consciousness you bring back this miniature movie ... and it will give you direction to help you create your own wonderful relationship ... your lover and yourself experiencing wonderful new, exciting experiences ... fully in tune.

As you start to return to full consciousness you feel stronger and wiser than before ... and you notice that the world is even more beautiful than you ever dreamed.'

The following are a set of inductions that can replace the above.

This next one is for couples to enjoy together. It will act as an inner cleansing element, clearing away the negative emotions and doubts and opening up the channels for happiness and positiveness. This very special induction was created by a very special, spiritual person on Langkawi, the Malaysian 'Island of Legends'.

Garden of Healing

'There is a door that leads you to a special place ... a place of healing ... you notice that the door is very grand ... and at the entrance to this beautiful door there is a person ... this very pleasant person is dressed very

modestly and comfortably ... you notice how peaceful he looks ... he greets you and asks you your purpose ... this surprises you ... and your answer also surprises you ... you contemplate your answer ... you notice the man is quite old and gives you the impression by his whole presence that he is very wise ... the wise old man says, "Beyond this door is a magnificent garden, a garden of healing, a garden of your dreams ... and in that garden is a brook ... the brook leads into a pool ... where you will cleanse yourself physically ... and beyond the pool a healing light ... a most wonderful healing light ... when you see this light you can sit down comfortably under it and relax even more."

He beckons and the door opens ... you enter the garden of healing ... a most beautiful garden ... you notice the scenery and it delights you ... and there ahead is the brook that runs into the pool ... as you walk to the pool you discard your garments ... garments of the past ... garments of negativity ... in your nakedness you immense yourself in the crystal clear and pure water ... washing away all your impurities ... cleansing yourself, preparing yourself ... all the negative feelings of fear are being washed away ... all sad feelings and unhappy feelings are being washed away ... all the feelings of inability are being cleansed from your body ... washed away ... all the unhappy feelings from the past that have inhibited you are leaving you ... being washed away ... by the purity of the crystal clear waters of the brook ... and you are absolutely fresh and clear like a newborn ... free of negativity but keeping all the positiveness you have experienced through life.

You are now ready to leave this special pool ... you now step out of the waters feeling fresh ... feeling pure

... feeling new ... take a moment to enjoy this wonderful experience ... [pause for 30 seconds] ... you are now ready to sit and relax under the beckoning warm glow of the healing light ... you approach it with a feeling of eagerness ... and anticipation.

This is a wonderful ... and healing light ... with a warm ... gentle glow ... this light will enter into your heart and bestow upon you the courage and the knowledge of true love ... you feel this new energy beginning to radiate through your body ... filling you with confidence ... and positive energy ... pure true love ... as the healing energy pulsates within you ... a new you is arising ... a better self ... a stronger self ... a confident self ... the positive you ... which has been lying dormant is now rushing to greet you ... a long lost friend ... enriching you with enthusiasm and peace ... and so many positive emotions ... and new feeling ... an awakening of a new radiance which emerges ... the embers of your true self ... of your heart and soul are now set aflame.

You hear yourself saying, "I am healed ... I feel great ... I radiate confidence ... every inch of my being ... my mind ... my body ... my spirit radiates energy ... dynamic and positive energy" ... you are the way you would like to be ... and now you are ready to embrace your partner and your relationship with an abundance of love ... and caring ... and bonding.'

Here is another beautiful, relaxing induction...

Colour my Heart

'As you begin your journey ... you enter a meadow ... it is the most beautiful meadow you have ever seen ... an expanse of flowers of many different hues ... you smell

the scent of your favourite flowers ... you see their colours and their shapes ... the wonderful smells are mixed with the dawn air ... for a moment you relax even more just thinking and experiencing the scents, textures and vision of your favourite flowers ... the smells intoxicate you with a calm and peaceful feeling ... a feeling of lightness soon fills your entire being ... in the distance you hear the gentle sound of a brook and trees slightly swaying in the soft breeze ... as you decide to walk toward the brook ... passing through the beautiful hues of colourful flowers ... two colours are more noticeable and these are your love and kindness colours ... as you reach the brook you bend to cup its crystal clear and cooling waters ... so clear ... so pure ... and as you quench your thirst with the sweet water ... you realize that its taste is so pleasant ... a subtle flavour ... so pure ... so refreshing ... so pleasing to your senses ... enriching you with its simple purity.

You step away from the cooling waters of the brook ... and you are attracted to a songbird ... a melodious songbird singing in the trees ... such a pretty and colourful bird ... with such a beautiful spontaneous song ... and with each melodious tone and pleasant feeling of freshness like a cool morning breeze, whispering pleasant tales of yesterday and glad tidings of tomorrow ... a feeling of contentment begins to run through your being ... a complete feeling of submission and as the sun rises and envelopes the field ... you experience total and complete peace and submission to the forces of the universe of true self ... of self-discovery and to the oneness of creation ... knowing you are in control of your destiny ... your actions can create happiness or despair ... the decision is easy for you to enjoy happiness and leave any despair in the past where it belongs ... you realize that life is filled with beauty for you to enjoy at your will.'

DEEPENERS

What is a Deepener?

A deepener is a suggestion given while the subject is in hypnosis for the purpose of attaining a deeper trance. The words used suggest that you will go deeper into hypnosis and allow the imagination to take the mind to an even deeper level of relaxation.

Why Do We Use It?

The purpose of a deepener is to make the subject completely relax, slowing down conscious thoughts and allowing suggestions to be accepted easily without too much interference from the logical, conscious part of the mind.

The deep trance does not have many benefits in advanced hypnotherapy, apart from when the subject needs to be anaesthetized for medical purposes. But it is wonderful for suggestion hypnosis. The feeling is that of deep relaxation and a peace of mind that is very comforting and secure. It helps you to focus your imagination better and an added advantage is that it shows how you can control your depth of trance.

How Do You Use a Deepener?

The stage hypnotist uses this technique to both entertain and put the subject quickly and deeper into hypnosis. He may say, *'When I snap my fingers you will go into a deeper sleep,'* and the subject immediately mimics a deep sleep. In fact, they are totally aware of everything that is going on but the subconscious is now in charge. It takes words literally and so is very precise in the actions it performs. If the subconscious is requested to act like a ballet dancer, which can happen with stage hypnosis, it will go into the memory banks and the person concerned will do an excellent imitation of a ballet dancer, pirouetting and all. The subject would normally be far too inhibited to do this consciously. Also, the memory files which incite such a brilliant performance aren't accessible to the conscious mind.

The Deepener

You can use a deepener *after* the induction and *before* the suggestion script (the suggestion scripts are covered in the next chapter). It is not absolutely necessary, though, and if you feel uncomfortable doing it, then don't include it in the hypnosis. It depends how you feel. You can't use this particular method at all if you are using a tape recorder, but if you are reading to your partner it is a good way to test how relaxed they are.

An example of a simple deepener would be to say: *'In a moment, when I snap my fingers, you will be doubly relaxed.'* Or, if your lover is sitting or lying down after the induction script, you just pick their arm up about 6 inches (15 cm) above their lap and say: *'When I count to three and drop your arm into your lap, you will be five times more relaxed.'* You then drop their arm into their lap. The mere act of dropping the arm triggers the instruction.

This is a fine way of finding out if your lover is indeed relaxed. Usually, the heavier the arm is, the deeper in relaxation they are. If the arm feels a little stiff, just shake it gently, like gently rocking a baby's cot, say, *'Let that arm become more relaxed now,'* and then drop it into their laps. Repeat the exercise with the other arm.

If their arm feels really stiff, or even light and floating, that, too, can be hypnosis. So don't presume that because the arm isn't doing what you expect that they are not relaxed enough. Just use it as a simple test.

Another example would be for you to say to your lover: *'In a moment I will ask you to open your eyes and I will count from one to three and then snap my fingers, and when I snap my fingers you will snap your eyes shut and then you will be doubly relaxed.'*

You then ask them to open their eyes, say, *'One, two, three,'* snap your fingers and as they close their eyes it will deepen their relaxation.

Finally ... there is a wonderful little trick to use for a re-shaping of your life. You need to do it daily for three weeks, so that it becomes a habit. First, you picture what you want. That's the hardest part, as most people don't know precisely what they want and find difficulty in being so detailed. You need to picture yourself doing whatever it is, feeling it and experiencing it. Then choose three words that describe your picture. Every morning as you awake, put yourself into hypnosis by picturing your muscles relaxing and bringing yourself to your garden bench. When you have practised the main progressive induction a few times, you will find it easy to get to your garden bench. Then just say those three words and they will act as a trigger.

This simple mind trick can make wonderful changes. You are programming your inner mind to what you want to achieve. This gives your subconscious something to work on. The great joy of this simple little technique is that you can change the words or re-programme your mind at any time because, who knows, your goals might change.

CHAPTER
THREE

Imagination is the doorway to the subconscious

The scripts in this chapter have been selected to help you in your search for full improvement. They vary from those aimed at bringing about a general building up of character to a special, all-important one for helping you to protect yourself from getting snared by a professional con artist or seducer. There is also a wide choice of sexual satisfaction suggestions that cover many problems, plus a wonderful 'blueprint' suggestion to spring clean your mind, whether you are in a relationship or not. To believe that your mind never needs a spring clean would be like never cleaning your house. The blueprint scripts were developed for the book, researched and reported in the case histories in Chapter 5, with outstanding results. It was interesting to note that the couples taking part did so as an experiment, each believing that their sex life could not possibly get better – in fact, it did in every case.

The main blueprint script, in my opinion, is a 'must' to clear out old doubts and negativity. I have had extraordinary results with it in just one group session. I hypnotized the couples together, suggesting that each listen and relax to both the *Love Blueprint for Men* and *Love Blueprint for Women* scripts. The inner mind will do the editing, picking out whichever one is relevant.

With the suggestion scripts, either read them to your lover or, if you decide to use a tape recorder, read more slowly and monotonously, highlighting certain words that are important to you. Talk much more slowly than you would if you were just reading to someone in the same room. When you are sitting comfortably or lying down, relaxing and waiting for the suggestions, you need a slow speed to allow you to pace your mind. Your mind will start to slow down as your breathing goes into the natural rhythm that you normally associate with sleep.

You can even mix and match the suggestions by borrowing words or whole paragraphs from the scripts below. Or you can start from scratch and create your own, using the examples and instructions and updating where necessary. Once the desired change in the behaviour pattern has been brought about you no longer need to keep repeating the suggestion.

HOW TO CREATE YOUR OWN SUGGESTIONS

It isn't difficult to create your own suggestions. But there are some important guidelines that you should follow:

- Use the present tense
  If you merely tell yourself in your suggestion that you will feel more confident and attach no time-scale to the instruction, your mind may take it literally and assume there is no hurry. It could put the programme into operation at some date in the future – say, in 10 years' time. Therefore, it is best to put a time limit on it or, to be on the safe side, use the present tense. For example: *'Every day from now on I feel more and more confident.'*

Or, as the principal aim of this book is to enable you to enhance your love life and enjoy a better relationship with your loved one, you could use sentences like: *'I feel more romantic and caring whenever I am with my partner.'*

- Be positive
Avoid using any negative words or phrases, such as 'I don't... ' or 'I am not...' or 'I would like to...' Instead, it is important to use phrases that are enthusiastic, determined and positively bristling with confidence and intent. Create a picture of what you *want* to do, rather than what you *don't want* to do.

   Imagine yourself as you want to be, not what you think you are at present. For instance, if you are having difficulties in a relationship, you might tell yourself: *'My relationship with my partner goes on getting better every day'* rather than: 'I would like to overcome the problems in my relationship.' The first suggests that your relationship is already good and can only go on getting better, while the second is negative by highlighting the fact that you have problems and doubts.

- Be specific
Stick to one problem at a time, rather than overload the mind with multiple demands. Don't have suggestions aimed at trying to stop smoking, lose weight, give up biting your nails and spice up your love life all in the same script. Also, be specific in your wording. 'I feel healthy' is too vague. *'I am recovering rapidly. With each new day I feel better and better'* would be more appropriate.

- Be detailed
Detail your new programme and affirm your desired activity by picturing it in your mind. Use the words that describe the picture as precisely as possible. Don't just say you 'want to be happy' because that isn't specific enough.

The subconscious needs direction because otherwise it might operate on an old programme and assume that what you want is something that made you happy five years ago! Describe what would make you happy right now. Detail it, whether it be how much money would make you happy, how successful you would like to be in your job, or whether you would like a new lover or want to make your present relationship even more fantastic.

- Be simple

Although the subconscious may be sophisticated, there is less chance of confusion if you keep the words simple. Treat your subconscious as if you were talking to a bright toddler.

- Use imaginative and exciting words

Exciting and imaginative words have much more energy and therefore your mind will react to them much more positively. Even if some words may seem old-fashioned to you now, the subconscious will take them literally and perhaps remember the energy they had for you in fairy stories when you were a child, exciting and stimulating your imagination. When formulating a suggestion to improve your sexual powers and relationship with your partner, use words like *'sensational'*, *'erotic'*, *'ecstasy'*, *'bliss'*, *'desire'* and *'satisfaction'*.

With the above guide, you can use one of the suggestions included in this chapter as a basis and change some of the wording to suit your individual needs. You may decide even to design the whole suggestion yourself. If you want to design one for someone else, you need to find out exactly what changes they are expecting to happen in their life and work the information around one of the basic scripts. There are no hard and fast rules in this department because every person – and every couple – is different. Some couples may prefer using lovey-dovey words and phrases, whilst others may relish turning each other on with the kind of explicit language you read in soft porn magazines. There is nothing wrong with either, as long as each partner is happy and completely in harmony with the other.

Here are the blueprint scripts.

Love Blueprint for Men
...for More Satisfying Relationships

'Holding hands is great but, as you know, there's more to life than just holding hands ... touching is one of the most basic forms of communication ... and when appropriate, it's also one of the most important forms of communication ... in fact where emotions are concerned, a genuine hug can say 1,000 words ... and usually far better than words.

Communicating through words alone is useful in a work environment ... where consistency and precision may be more important than feelings ... people, however, are not machines ... and our most rewarding relationships are those where we can express our feelings ... in fact, the quality of all our relationships ... improves as we learn to relate to people, as people.

You are here because you have chosen to improve your relationships ... it's one of the best decisions of your life ... and you recognize the increased happiness created by understanding ... what makes people feel at ease ... most people, given the choice, would prefer to be happy rather than sad ... and to make things easier ... we tend to choose friends who also like to be happy ... unpopular people tend to be those who wallow in their problems ... or derive pleasure by making others unhappy ... these people often attract illness and bad luck ... you have wisely chosen to have healthy relationships.

From now on, you always remember that people would prefer to see your best side ... because your best side is who you really are ... we always see people at their worst ... when they get defensive ... when we get defensive, we're no better ... gone are the days when you'd invite unhelpful or disruptive people into your life ... the best way to greet new people is with a friendly attitude and to take each moment as it comes ... no matter what someone looks like ... no matter who they may remind you of ... no matter who they sound like ... anyone can be your friend ... knowing this makes your body language more approachable and makes you look more friendly ... the more friendly you look, the more people will trust you ... the more you socialize, the easier you find it to recognize people who are trustworthy and considerate ... you do this by listening carefully to what they say ... and by observing the way they treat others ... and by the way they treat you.

The more time you spend with these people ... the more you recognize your own worth ... you enjoy spending time with them ... and they enjoy spending time with you ... quite naturally, you understand people's likes and dislikes ... your listening skills continuously improve and bring ever greater rewards ... you now find that you can introduce people you feel to be compatible together.

Relationships are the same the whole world over ... if you are compatible and you trust each other, there is a basis for a relationship ... after that, everything hinges on the honesty each of you has about your feelings ... the more honest you are ... the happier you are ... you never do things just trying to please someone ... because by living a lie, you know you only delay the inevitable ... saying what you feel avoids you bottling up your feelings ... when you talk about your emotions, you assert yourself naturally ... you find no need to raise your voice and you explain yourself in a calm but purposeful way ... this way, your partner recognizes the importance of what you're saying ... and finds it easy to listen to you ... in return, you do the same for them and your relationships thrive.

Touching is a natural part of our body language, which communicates directly with our emotions ... whilst body language is a whole language in itself ... you already know when someone looks comfortable and when someone does not ... just as you like your space to be respected ... you are both aware and respectful of other people's space.

All relationships are built in trust and all parties must be fully consenting ... you make sure you always check how comfortable people are around you ... you do this by observing their body language ... and by talking to them ... and then making the appropriate adjustments to the way that you relate to the person that you are with ... whenever you're in doubt ... you mention it gently ... so that you can both talk about your feelings ... and begin to feel comfortable again.

You enjoy having relaxed and meaningful relationships ... finding that this is the healthiest environment in which trust can grow ... intimacy is achieved as both of you progressively drop the barriers that prevent you from being totally honest with each other ... all your relationships benefit from your new behaviour ... which also brings a more profound understanding of people and their desires ... it also allows you to be more honest with your own.

Quite naturally ... through healthy communication ... there will be someone who really relates to you ... someone whose company you really enjoy ... comfortable with them, you are now able to explore a greater level of intimacy ... you know that there's no urgency ... and that the relationship has its own pace ... all the time you are able to communicate your feelings ... and are also in touch with the feelings of your partner ... our bodies love to be touched ... that's why we're made the way we are ... you acknowledge that there are few pleasures in life greater than being intimate with someone you trust and care for.

You enjoy taking your time and understand that there's no correct way to do anything ... you just listen to your heart and do what feels right ... it's like a journey ... you could take the motorway ... but you choose to take the scenic route ... you're not just interested in getting there ... you want to savour every moment ... really enjoying the journey ... you allow yourself lots of time and find out what your partner's likes are ... your partner deeply appreciates your tenderness ... and the rewards are ... really touching ... you sense and feel love like never before ... and the sexual expression of this passion flows through you with ease ... you experiment, take breaks ... and find it easy to keep your sense of fun ... loving has never been easier ... rich in love, you blossom ... and every day your life just gets better ... and better.'

Love Blueprint for Women
...for More Satisfying Relationships

'The reason that you are here is because you've recognized that you're now ready to make changes in your

life ... *changes that alter the way that you experience the world ... changes that enable you to see yourself in a more positive light ... changes ... so that you can truly enjoy your experiences ... not only is it time to change the way you perceive yourself ... it's also time to free yourself of the unhelpful labels ... labels that may be associated with some of the sensations that you feel ... labels that limit your enjoyment and prevent you from living your life to the full ... the words "good" and "bad" are nothing more than labels ... generally when we get what we want, we call it "good" ... when we don't get what we expect, we call it "bad" ... good and bad are only labels because they merely reflect our perceptions and our expectations.*

Our perceptions are just our opinions and these can be wrong ... we all make mistakes ... the more you forgive others ... the more you forgive yourself ... and the more others forgive you. From now on, you're never concerned by right and wrong ... instead you consider appropriateness ... *you understand that feelings of love may be wonderful ... but that physically displaying these passionate feelings may be appropriate in some places ... whilst inappropriate in others ... at no point does love ever become bad ... sex and romance are activities that are part of the loving experience ... and they, too, can never be bad ... other people's opinions are just that ... opinions ... these opinions are formed around the labels ... that these people have unconsciously chosen to limit their lives ... their opinions are their problems ... and you don't lose any of your energy worrying about other people's problems ... you take them with a pinch of salt ... some opinions, however, are helpful feedback ... and you'll know in your heart if they are ... because you always listen to your heart ... no matter what may have been said ... or done ... in the past, you are now free ... no more can an old hurt affect the way you live your life now ... you direct your life ... no one else ... you are not a victim ... you are free ... no more could you allow someone to hold an influence over you ... because you know that by your birthright ... you are equal to anybody on this planet ... no one is better than you ... no one is less than you ... no one can take your energy away ... only you can give it away ... you fundamentally understand ... that you ... and only you ... are responsible for your well-being ... you make your life what it is.*

Gone are the days spent trying to live your life by other people's rules ... gone are the days spent trying to please everyone else ... the only person that you set out to please is yourself ... you are pleased when you know ... that your pleasure did not come at someone else's expense ... for you to win, others do not have to lose ... you understand the value of living without sacrifice ... you are special ... you're alive ... you have been granted the gift of life ... and that's the whole gift, including all that comes with it ... fun, friends, fulfilment, love ... and, of course, sex.

Quite simply, without sex, none of us would be here ... thankfully, because it's so enjoyable ... it's also one of the main reasons that we're here ... not just to make babies, but to experience joy ... what makes living so amazing is that not only is it so great to be alive ... but that by being alive ... we are able to experience love and sex ... deeply, you understand that life really is sweet.

Sensations change continuously ... it's a fact of life ... some sensations that you once didn't enjoy can become exquisite ... anything from looking at a painting ... to being tickled ... can now become truly sensational ...

you are always in charge of your body ... and the experience cannot be limited by anyone else's opinions ... you ... and only you ... can be the judge of whether you're enjoying yourself ... nobody else's judgement counts ... their labels are worthless in your experience ... you only concern yourself with what feels good to you ... and when would be an appropriate time to do something about it ... maybe straightaway, maybe later ... whichever feels right for you is what's best for you ... from now on, you instinctively know whether a situation is appropriate ... in keeping with all things in life ... it's when no one feels hurt ... consent is the key ... everything is possible between consenting adults and without it nothing happens ... without your consent, nothing can happen to you.

From now on, you are the sole ruler of your body ... nothing can happen to you against your will ... when anything in your life is unpleasurable ... you simply say "Stop" ... and mean it ... your happiness needs no one's approval ... so when you say "Stop" ... they know that you mean it ... this is now your normal behaviour ... at all times of your everyday life ... people can't help but think of you as attractive ... fun ... and great company ... but certainly not somebody who could be pushed around ... instantly people treat you with more respect ... because you now treat yourself with more respect ... people follow your lead ... no more do you have any time for people who don't respect women ... or other people's feelings ... it's your life and you choose who you wish to spend time with.

The men who are attracted to you ... see you as an equal ... they see you as someone rather special ... someone who has self-worth ... the type of men that you attract ... now have self-worth ... like attracts like

... from now on, all your relationships are based on respect ... trust ... and love ... in these relationships, tenderness feels completely natural ... it's understood that there's no rush because every moment becomes even more exciting as it's savoured ... you enjoy giving lingering caresses ... as much as you enjoy receiving them ... in love there are no rules ... only consent.

Without constraints, you are free to enjoy your body to the full ... relaxed at all times and always without trying to please ... you are now far more aware of the sensations that course through your body ... far more aware of the sensations flying through your mind ... so much so that in your love-making ... all of your awareness ... is completely absorbed by the exquisite feelings that you're experiencing ... it's as if each sensation has a note that plays inside you ... and the different parts of your body play different notes ... completely relaxed, you gradually become more ... and more ... aware of the melody released from within you ... and the harmony between the two of you ... now, as you truly let go ... trusting yourself to the feelings that have guided star-crossed lovers for thousands of years ... you, too ... begin to sense the freedom and the music that flood into our lives ... when we stop thinking and allow our hearts to sing ... in every moment of your passionate sex ... all that you sense ... are your sensational feelings and your rapture ... quite naturally, your partner feels it too without a word being said ... as you let go ... you realize ... that you're letting go of nothing ... and in return ... the reward for your trust ... is bliss.'

For the Over-Sexed

'What's the problem with being over-sexed?' cynics might ask. However this script is aimed at those who may think they are having a wonderful sex life by sleeping around and constantly moving on to a new partner. In reality, they don't know they're missing the shared joy of a genuine relationship. They may be getting oodles of sex but have no real love in their life – and how sad it all looks to a well-adjusted person. It is usually a symptom of low self-esteem. The person who is over-sexed is usually disassociated from reality, not realizing they are not feeling true pleasure. So, like the drug addict, they have to have more and more to satisfy another urge that has little to do with sex.

'We're all creatures of habit ... until we recognize our habits ... some habits only cause us a little harm ... and some habits ... though once useful ... have now outgrown their use ... causing us unwanted behaviour ... we get into habits by repeating certain activities ... that make us feel good in some way.

When we're young, sexual prowess is sometimes mistaken for status ... when this is the case, we're having sex to boost our ego rather than to satisfy a real physical urge ... in a sense, we have a need ... need to be seen to perform ... we're trying to prove something ... and it's not our love.

No more ... from now on, you recognize yourself as complete ... and accept yourself ... feeling good in your skin ... you don't need anyone's approval ... you're great as you are ... you've got nothing to prove ... in fact, you're aware that when someone tries to prove something about themselves ... it's because they themselves don't believe it ... having sex is easy ... but making love is not a performance ... you recognize that you prefer quality ... to quantity ... you understand that people who become obsessed by quantity are either doing it to impress ... or because they're not really experiencing the full effect of their involvement ... As an adult, you know that only teenagers would boast about how many times they managed to perform ... you're far more interested in savouring and experiencing sex ... fully.

Now, you choose to participate fully in your love-making ... allowing yourself the time and the gentleness to become truly satisfied ... rather than only experience the sex in a few parts of your body ... now you can sense all the feelings coursing through all of your body ... in the past, you didn't make the most of what you had ... no more ... no more are you worried that the grass may be greener elsewhere ... you get the greatest satisfaction by making the most of what you've got.

Never again do you have sex ... just to take your mind off something that you don't want to think about ... you know that the problem doesn't go away ... you deal with your problems methodically and openly and you understand that you prefer to make love with a clear mind ... because your mind is then free to really enjoy itself ... every single second ... every single touch.'

Attracting the Right Mate – Clearing the Channels

'Everyone has a soul-mate ... unfortunately most humans experience difficulty in seeing someone's soul ... so the most important thing about our true partner ... is invisible to our eyes ... all our lives we've been conjuring images in our minds ... images about how

our partner should look ... some people may even get it right ... but the truth is ... it's not about looks ... it's much deeper than that ... some people spend all their lives chasing looks ... and personalities ... choosing not to recognize the deeper character of the person that they're with ... until it becomes obvious that needy love is blind.

Recognizing this, you have chosen to make yourself ready to meet your right mate ... the two important things that you do to clear the channels ... are to free yourself of any emotional attachments other than friends and family ... and also to free yourself of your limiting beliefs ... about yourself or your life ... you understand that while there's someone in your heart ... you're not open to recognize your soul-mate ... if deep down you know that the person in your heart is not your soul-mate ... then you have the strength to set them free ... that way you're free to meet your soul-mate ... and they're free to meet theirs.

When your heart is free ... you are open to meet your true partner ... take your time ... it's not a matter of having to choose ... the right person will make themselves totally obvious to you ... as long as you don't keep looking for them ... this only pushes them away ... the universe will bring them to you quite naturally ... all you have to do is enjoy your life being you ... you are complete without a partner ... you do not need a partner to make you whole ... until you know this, you will find it difficult to recognize your soul-mate ... you understand this and are now prepared to meet your partner ... by clearing your heart ... soul-mates meet ... when and only when ... each of the people involved has evolved ... to the stage where they recognize their own beauty and completeness ... in

other words ... when they learn to love themselves ...
only then do they truly know ... that they are worthy
of love ... until this happens in our life, all our relationships are learning grounds ... where we get to
know ourselves ... It is best to really understand this ...
or you might end up marrying someone ... just because
you can!

To truly accept yourself is to recognize your life as
limitless ... that, ultimately, you are allowed to be
happy ... it's not about having fabulous wealth ... or
doing a wonderful job ... you deeply understand that
we are human beings ... not human doings ... money ...
and jobs ... do not ensure your happiness ... being
happy being you ... is the only thing that can do this.

Systematically, you free yourself of all your limiting
beliefs ... this is not a life of sacrifice ... this is not a life
of compromises ... this is a life of conscious choices ...
consciously, you understand your true worth ... unconsciously, we allow ourselves to be unhappy ... you,
quite brilliantly, have chosen to be conscious of your
existence ... of your right to have your cake ... and eat it
... and of your right to be ... Now you are ready ...
allow it to happen naturally.'

Attracting a Sexually Compatible Partner

'You are now attracting into your life people who are
sexually compatible with you ... from these people, one
in particular stands out as being a person ... with whom
you are willing to develop a close bond ... you find
yourself able to open up to this person ... and your
revealing your vulnerability allows them to come
towards you in intimacy and love ... as this mutual

intimacy blossoms ... you find each other more and more sexually attractive and compatible.

As you explore the miracle of your own and your partner's sexuality ... you know that any conflict ... that arises between you ... is a gift to enable you to join together in love ... and reach an even higher level of mutual understanding and support ... in fact, you welcome the conflict as being a natural part of the process of moving towards each other ... and an opportunity to explore each other in wonder and love ... you recognize that any aspect of your partner that you want to criticize or attack ... simply mirrors a part of you that you have dissociated from ... as you reconnect with your partner ... so does your ability to show them your wounds and to receive their love ... you recognize that any time you experience your partner as attacking you is simply their call for love ... and you respond with ever greater compassion and warmth ... you know that together you can resolve any difficulty ... and that the path you tread together is a journey towards realizing the Godhead in yourself and in each other.

You also know that your time together ... is exactly the right time for you to be with each other ... and to learn the lessons that you have for each other ... then, when this time is complete and the lessons learned ... you can let each other go in love and gratefulness ... for the gifts that you have received and given ... let them go without any attachment ... even to their memory ... so that when it is right for you to be with another partner ... you have created the space to allow that person in ... and the right partner will be there for you ... and, of course, you are always free to recommit yourself to the partner you already have ... at any time.'

This next script is for the person who has perhaps married for the wrong reasons – maybe for financial gain or purely for emotional security – and is not sexually attracted to their spouse. Hypnosis can allow you to see the beauty in the person you are with.

Turning a Frog into a Prince

'The person you have chosen for your life-long partner ... may not look the way you want them to ... but you begin to see them in a new light ... in your mind, when making love ... you turn them into a fantasy playmate ... perhaps they look like your favourite movie star ... features which were unpleasant to you seem different ... interesting ... a part of their character ... you find it easy to turn them into a special playmate ... a part of your inner self that creates images ... to bring you full excitement ... your lover becomes your favourite heart-throb ... as they love you ... embrace you ... you feel excited ... wonderful ... and the chemistry between you is turned on ... every part of your body ... reacts and tingles.

Your body knows how to be turned on ... you have used your mind to activate this easy ... natural ... procedure when you have masturbated ... your inner mind creates a wonderful situation so you can have orgasms with your lover ... and what is even more exciting ... you can exude love and attraction ... and electrifying energy that they willingly pick up and in turn excites them ... creating a wonderful timing that is perfect for you both ... so you are both satisfied simultaneously ... climaxing because you have directed your lover with your own mind ... directed them with love and giving to receive.

All you know is that you follow your body ... what it

wants to do ... and you know your lover has nothing to be jealous about ... as your playmate is only your strategy for creating the perfect environment for sexual pleasure and romance.'

The next two scripts are for those who have been in broken relationships and want to rid themselves of any emotional baggage they may be carrying around with them as a result.

When You Have Loved and Lost

'Every trauma, problem and obstacle that has happened in the past has been put to use ... in building up your strength and your character ... to allow you to begin to see your future more clearly ... more positively that ever before ... your emotions now begin to settle down ... the anger, the frustration and the hurt you felt before ... which got in the way of your decision-making ... are now back in their correct places ... leaving valuable information ... from experience ... that will enable you to draw better and more constructive conclusions ... the emotions settle down ... no longer on the surface ... no longer in the way of your thinking clearly ... they have served their purpose and because your mind is now stronger ... clearer ... and more positive than before ... you begin to feel the benefits ... your confidence is stronger and healthier ... you believe in yourself ... as a person ... and a woman/man ... you enjoy your new respect and no longer carry hurt around with you ... like a damp bundle of dirty washing ... instead you are proud of yourself and your new attitude ... your attitude is no longer a problem.

You realize that if people say hurtful things it is

because they have a problem ... and are frustrated ...
you can understand that the remarks and the actions ...
that would have hurt you in the past may be a retaliation ... retaliation for a hurt they were experiencing ...
it does not prevent you from examining yourself to
check whether it is your fault ... but this time you are
able to do so in a constructive way ... and you are able
to work on your faults and weaknesses to enable you to
grow and ... be happy ... and contented.

Your inner mind ... works at building and strengthening your weaknesses ... the weaknesses that have
caused you so much mental anguish ... resulting in a
wonderful peace of mind ... as your emotions settle ...
new, positive emotions now come to the surface ...
replacing the old, useless, negative emotions ... happiness ... a sense of humour and a love of life replace ...
anxiety ... hurt ... and anger.

The bad habit of worrying is minimized ... it is unproductive and destructive ... because now your mind is
open to positive thoughts and you find that you visualize
yourself easily and often as happy ... smiling ... ready to
enjoy the wonderful experiences your life has to offer ...
this very action indicates to your subconscious ... your
inner mind ... what you wish ... and your subconscious
will be instructed by the language of visualization to
follow your wishes ... resulting in your happiness.'

The End of a Relationship

'You are a confident ... self-assured ... independent
person ... fully able to satisfy your own requirements
yourself without being dependent on or affected by
another person ... your self-love is more than adequate

... it lets you be perfectly at home with yourself ... you are fully aware of your own sexuality and recognize your abundant ability to love and be loved ... you have cleared all of your past incompatibilities ... and are totally at home with the past ... knowing that it has no hold over you anymore ... you are extremely happy when you see your previous partner is following their own dreams ... when you see them ... they will remind you how much freedom and independence you now hold ... now you can focus all your energies into fulfilling your ambitions and dreams ... allowing space for someone who can give you all that you could wish for and more.

You feel stronger ... healthier ... more vibrant and full of self-love ... your energy is increased as you open up to all the possibilities available to you ... this new-found source of energy and your greater sense of awareness allow you to feel more ... see ... more ... enjoy all that you experience as if for the first time ... your confidence is so strong ... you are at home with yourself ... whether alone in bed at night ... or out meeting new people ... when you prepare for sleep ... you look forward to luxuriating in the expanse of your own bed ... feeling exhilarated of being able to do anything you want ... without answering to any other.

Your self-assurance completely obliterates all those tiny fears that may have plagued you in the past ... you feel secure and safe, knowing that your environment is strongly protected by its powerful energy.'

Indecision and Change of Mind

'In this beautiful state of pure relaxation ... you feel an inner glow of contentment because you instinctively know that you have the ability to decide which changes are most beneficial to you ... in fact, the ability for you to make decisions just flows from within ... so automatically ... that you become filled with extra confidence and energy ... this in turn enables you to accomplish more and the result is that you feel good about yourself ... you find it easy to be able to imagine yourself making decisions, whether big or small ... it puts a smile on your face because it is such a lovely feeling to be sure ... when you have a choice to make, the answer just tumbles to your lips ... your mind is clear ... alert ... responsive.

You can see yourself now, talking with others ... and giving the answers to questions raised ... the conversation flows along beautifully ... others so admire your ability to make decisions ... this is just one aspect that draws others to you ... you acquire a feeling of personal power ... decisions in your business ventures are an easy task for you now ... you are sure of yourself ... you know your mind has the ability to lead you in the right direction and ultimately to the perfect conclusion ... you can now trust in this process working for you at all times ... so life becomes fun ... you are the master decision-maker.'

Jealousy

'At last, you have taken control of your life ... by choosing to slay the green-eyed monster called jealousy

... *many of us have learned to be jealous from other people ... who used it as a cheap way of showing passion ... you know that passion is an intense energy and that jealousy is a misuse of this energy.*

Put simply, you can only feel jealous of someone else ... by undervaluing what you have ... this usually comes about when people play the comparison game ... it is a game you're guaranteed to lose ... because then ... the grass is always greener somewhere else.

By being jealous, your actions indicate to your partner ... that there is someone you feel might be better suited to them than you ... nowadays, you understand that jealousy pushes people away ... jealousy is repulsive ... jealousy is not a feeling based on love ... it is a feeling based on possessiveness and control ... love is the magical binding force that makes people want to spend time together ... it only thrives when each person is free.

You know that it's impossible to hold someone who is in love ... love is a natural phenomenon ... it's probably the wonder that all other wonders have been built on ... and that includes your existence ... you are here because of love ... to fight this is to be at odds with nature ... whilst you are trying to control someone, you cannot truly feel their love ... by setting them free, you can then see if they would naturally choose you ... if they don't come back ... you are then free to meet the right partner for you ... either way ... you move one step closer to your heart ... from now on you recognize jealousy as a waste of time and a waste of your life ... instead, you choose to live in love ... a state where everyone is free.'

Jealousy is a negative emotion and can become active within a relationship even if the person now experiencing it has never done so before. The above suggestion can help clear it, but here is another effective trick that you can use after the suggestion while you are still in hypnosis.

The first step is to imagine that you are going to bring forward a shape which represents the jealousy. It can be anything – a square, a ring or any other shape at all. Then, when you have the shape or object in your imagination, check what it is made of. At this point you may have to create what it is made of in your mind. Make sure you imagine both the shape and what it is made of before you go on to the next step.

Now imagine how you can get rid of it. Any method of dispensing with the offending shape or object is fine, the more bizarre the better in fact. You can drench it in acid, set it alight or blow it up, but just make sure you obliterate it totally. You are wiping out the jealousy, banishing it from your inner mind forever.

This is a wonderfully powerful tool and a similar method has been used very effectively with terminally ill cancer patients. If you don't visualize, it is more difficult but still can be done using your own method of imagination. I know this because, as I have mentioned earlier, I do not picture things at all and, yet I have used this method on myself very effectively. I used it for getting rid of a woolly feeling in my mind when I had my memory loss.

Unfaithfulness

'In relationships, people can be unfaithful for many reasons ... but one thing is for certain ... and that is that both partners play a part in the events that unfold ...

what you must always remember is that if someone is totally centred ... happy ... enjoying their life to the full and being themselves ... then their partner would not be attracted to anyone else and would not leave them ... when we allow ourselves to behave as less than we really are ... our real worth is no longer seen by our partner ... and eventually they may be tempted to look elsewhere ... it's your job to keep your light burning bright ... the world does not owe you a living.

If you are the partner who looked elsewhere ... don't feel completely guilty ... accept that it happened for a reason ... you can learn from it and your relationship can now be made even stronger ... the fact that you've chosen to return to your partner means that you've found a redeeming light in them ... that makes them outshine the person you were recently attracted to.

If your partner has been unfaithful, do not hold any grudges ... seeking revenge will only hurt you more in the long run ... by being adult about it, you'll see that there's a gift for you ... inadvertently, your partner has created a space for you to grow in ... a place for you to heal yourself from the point of sacrifice that you'd reached ... to them you no longer looked like the whole person that they fell in love with ... the fact that they've chosen to return to you is a sign that they recognize that you've grown during the course of this experience, so a new relationship can start ... this time with better communication ... both of you acknowledge that the communication between you was not working properly ... sometimes it was because one partner was not saying how they really felt ... and sometimes it was because they weren't listening properly to each other ... for listening is loving.

In any relationship, no matter how good the

chemistry ... no matter how beautiful the people are ... without communication, the relationship will not survive ... your desire to be together is felt by how much you love to communicate with your partner ... it's a measure of your love ... every time you meet your relationship changes and grows ... every conversation ... every touch ... every event is another stepping-stone in your relationship's growth ... by truly expressing the feelings in your heart, you give your partner a greater opportunity to understand you ... and to show their feelings to you ... expressing yourself sets you free ... free to be honest and free to feel.

Handled in an adult manner ... unfaithfulness can be one of the richest growth phases that a relationship can experience ... it's not about blame ... blaming is for children ... as an adult you accept and move forward with grace ... to accept the events without blame is to accept your partner and yourself ... in this life you are each other's teacher and guide ... that's the reason that you've been brought together.

Partners reflect each other ... and our partner can show us more about ourselves than anyone else ... every day we are alive to learn ... stubbornness is a refusal to learn and a refusal to grow ... you wouldn't want to stay with a partner who refused to learn and to grow ... and nor would your partner ... people who like to be stubborn can also expect to be lonely.

From now on, you'd rather learn ... than try to be right all the time ... you hold no grudges against your partner and no adverse feelings about yourself regarding your past actions ... from now on you only live for today ... the fact is that you're back together and committed to your relationship ... this time you chose to communicate fully and to stay responsible for yourself at all times ... loving yourself is loving your partner ... and loving your partner is loving yourself.'

Anger Release

'Because you want to live a happy and harmonious life with other people ... and enjoy good health ... physically ... and emotionally ... you have a feeling of peace and tolerance with everyone ... you realize that each personality is a product of heredity and experience ... you know that if you had been born as someone else and had lived through their experiences, you would act exactly as they do ... therefore, you accept others as they are ... and when they do things you disapprove of, the only emotions you feel are sympathy and understanding ... you are in complete control of your emotions at all times ... even under what others believe to be stressful conditions.

This gives you a feeling of great satisfaction ... you feel and express only the good, healthy emotions ... of love ... kindness ... sympathy and tolerance to others ... you love other people for their good qualities ... and you forgive them for the acts you disapprove of ... because you know they are doing what you would do with their same body, experiences and level of awareness.

From now on you are able to get in touch with your pent-up emotions and deal with them in a constructive manner ... whenever these negative feelings appear you find ways of redirecting them in some acceptable way ... all your hidden personal reasons for the angry ... hostile ... feelings may or may not communicate to your conscious mind ... the awareness that is communicated to your conscious mind is dealt with in a constructive ... practice and sensible way.

Whatever still remains of these feelings that are no longer serving any useful purpose ... are got rid of ... dumped by your subconscious ... put into your mind's waste bin and disintegrated ... dissipated ... replaced by positive, wonderful feelings ... leaving you quite free to get on with and enjoy your life ... no longer hindered by negativity ... from now on your mind always starts to process all your guilt feelings ... it gradually accepts that because you are only human you have human failings ... your subconscious mind finds ways to discard and come to terms with those guilty feelings you have no control over ... those feelings in the past that nothing can be done about ... you shake them off completely ... and at all levels ... your mind works on ways you can get rid of other guilty feelings by taking some action ... to change what can be changed.

From now on, you quickly recover your sense of humour and your sense of proportion ... you feel better and more optimistic, with renewed energy ... you dwell on the things you have to be grateful for ... happy memories and things to look forward to ... from now on you won't get nearly so upset about remarks or hurtful incidents ... these have less and less effect on you ... you realize that they aren't really intended to upset or hurt you ... they just won't bother you anymore ... things just won't be able to get under your skin so much ... inwardly you are much stronger day by day ... much better to withstand hurts and disappointments ... far ... far less vulnerable ... than before.'

The 'Con' Script

Sadly, there are some people who always seem to pick the wrong person in their relationships, perhaps because they are naïve, vulnerable, lonely or simply looking for someone to give them affection. These people are easy prey for the sharks out there – and there are a lot of them, of both sexes! For example, the other person may be married or establishing a relationship or friendship for an ulterior motive.

So this script is for those unfortunates who keep on being conned and want to put a halt to their constant stream of unsatisfactory relationships.

'You are a confident ... happy ... intelligent person ... you have an innate integrity and honesty and are open to people ... knowing you are this wonderful ... human being ... you instinctively attract similar people to you ... it is easy for you to discern when people are not being honest with you ... it will stand out immediately and your natural protection will automatically put you on guard and make you wary ... without effort, you will see through anyone who is not what they appear and their true motives will instantly become clear ... this intuitive knowledge will enable you to easily defuse any manipulation they attempt against your person ... quickly and firmly turning it back on themselves.

Without requiring any deviousness from yourself ... you will find yourself maintaining your centred being ... holding true to yourself ... and allowing yourself to remain a happy ... loving ... and open person, while deflecting any manipulation by another person for their own ends ... your incredible, well-developed intuition will instantly determine whether someone is attempting to rip you off ... *your naturally well-developed sense of character will allow you to assess whether someone is worthy of your attentions ... and the people who are not what they seem will immediately become obvious ... and you will automatically make sure they are incapable of taking anything from you.*

This remarkable ability you have ... will apply to all things ... and all people ... you can tell if something is worth buying ... or worth doing ... and if it is right for you ... you revel in this natural ability and every time you become aware of it working for you ... you will be filled with a sense of well-being ... and confident ... making it easier ... and easier ... to make correct, competent and permanent decisions.'

Shyness

'*You have found that your subconscious is clearing the channels of your confidence ... allowing that natural self-confidence to work more easily ... and more comfortably each day ... it becomes as natural as breathing ... and you never have to think about it ... it just happens ... you feel secure and comfortable with yourself ... you enjoy speaking to people because you like to meet new people ... and make new friends ... what might have been difficult in the past is now easy ... your future looks bright and friendly ... from now on you feel comfortable with new people whom you choose to talk to and mix with ... it adds the spice ... to the rich tapestry of life ... chance encounters often lead to fun ... and sometimes ... to very special relationships.*

You realize it takes two to make a conversation ... and you also realize that most people find it difficult to start a conversation ... you realize that all you need is your friendly smile to break the ice ... a simple "Hello" and a confidence in yourself which is always attractive to another person ... a shy approach can be very off-putting and makes the other person nervous ... so you find that you now feel confident when you are in other people's company and you enjoy being friendly.

Because you have been shy in the past it has given you the great skill of being a good listener ... and that is very attractive to other people ... people love to be listened to and you are able to do this with ease whenever you want to ... but this time it is for the right reasons ... not because you are too shy to talk ... but because you are interested in people ... and you find out so much about the person you are interested in making friends with.

You find you won't need clever chat-up lines or witty responses ... people like to meet real people ... people like you ... they want to meet your personality ... not rehearsed speeches or lines ... it is important to remember that the most special social skill is the ability to listen ... because everybody loves a good listener ... a listener puts people at ease ... and you have had a lot of practice at this skill ... and now you can use it when you want to instead of it being a necessity.

Your subconscious has stored all the information that it has picked up from interesting and caring people ... all this information is at hand ... you can be your own role model ... you have all the information that allows you to be the person you want to be ... and your subconscious allows you to be this person ... by allowing you to enjoy a confidence that is your right ... you look forward to a happy and fulfilling life as a confident person ... each time you relax and use self-hypnosis it triggers your subconscious ... to gather up all the doubts

and negativity that were in the way of you being a confident person ... you don't have to try ... your subconscious works for you ... giving you a spring clean ...
ridding you of all the doubts and hurts that you have
experienced in the past ... you develop a sense of
humour and realize that life is not meant to be difficult
... and is as easy and comfortable as you want it to be.'

Stopping Swearing

Some people have difficulty in making and maintaining
relationships because they have fallen into a habit of using
bad language, which others do not find in the slightest bit
attractive.

'You are well educated, with an excellent vocabulary ...
strongly persuasive ... eloquent and articulate ... without
the need to swear ... when you get irritated ... angry or
upset ... there is no need to use offensive swear words ...
take time to express your thoughts and feelings in a positive way ... think for a few moments of words that will
not upset ... or offend your partner ... or people who are
important to your partner ... and use these words in the
future ... you do not want the reputation of being a foul-
mouthed ... ignoramus ... it does not match the image
you are seeking ... it is not in the least sexy or attractive.
    Swearing is not natural ... it is a very bad habit that
we pick up from others around us ... usually when we
are too young to know any better ... you have the ability to lose this very bad habit quickly ... and easily ... by
exchanging swear words with inoffensive words ... and
explanations that will not upset ... or offend yourself or
others ... you no longer have the need or desire to swear

... swearing is not for adults ... swearing is for people who have not yet learned that it looks ... and sounds ... silly ... and immature.

You may think that some people don't mind it ... but do you really know who does and who doesn't? ... now, to be absolutely sure of the image you want, you no longer need or desire to swear.'

Sarcastic Trait

This is for the person who risks wrecking their relationships by allowing a sarcastic streak to surface, perhaps in nasty and cutting remarks to their partner.

'Because you want to enjoy your relationship and have peace within yourself ... you find you can now deal with negative emotions in a more constructive way ... you no longer need to change everything that is positive or nega-tive ... to negative ... that is precisely what you are doing when you are being sarcastic ... it may not be so disrup-tive to you ... but it hurts the ones you love and care for ... it hurts them because all negative words have a reac-tion in the body ... and constant use can start a programme of self-doubt ... look at it through the eyes of the person you are firing your sarcasm at ... these nega-tive, sarcastic words are being spoken by a person that is important to you ... even though you may know outwardly that they do not necessarily mean it ... the words give an inner reaction ... and the more regularly they are said, the more they have the dreadful possibility of creating an unwanted programme of self-doubt ... would you like that to happen to you? ... or, more impor-tant, do you want that to happen to the one you love?

You know that getting rewards or achieving a wonderful love is damaged by your sarcasm ... hurting others through your sarcasm will only hurt you more ... it only shows your weaknesses ... insecurity and immaturity on your part.

From now on you know that you will use the strategy for sarcasm in a more constructive way ... changing to enhancing your relationship ... allowing your partner to feel good ... so they can be proud of themselves and of you ... they can hold their head up and know they will not be put down ... made to feel embarrassed in public or even in private ... knowing that you care so much ... enabling them to respect themselves and in turn respect you.

You find that now you can congratulate others on their achievements and gains ... sharing their happiness and you feel good about doing this ... you now earn your respect ... curt remarks have no place in your life ... they are flushed away down the sewers by your inner mind, leaving you free to express yourself ... in a pleasant, loving and acceptable way ... liking yourself every time you do it ... from now on you quickly recover your sense of humour and feel better and more optimistic ... with revived energy ... to be the new you ... the new you will be a person you will be proud of.'

For Good Health and a Wonderful Body

'I am at home in my body ... I am very comfortable there ... I appreciate my body ... it is fit and strong and full of joy ... my body and mind are working harmoniously together ... I have a dynamic ... successful and powerful partnership between my mind and my body

... I take care of myself because I respect myself ... and in respecting myself I am sending out the right energies that attract the people I want ... and who are good for me ... I attract people who respect themselves ... I am confident in my subconscious to send out the right signals so I can enjoy a relationship ... if ... and when ... the time is right.

Every day, as my mind becomes stronger ... my body becomes stronger ... as I become stronger and healthier ... stress and anxiety begin to vanish ... the food I eat is highly nutritious and of great benefit to me ... I find I prefer good healthy food and my mind and body work in harmony ... to instruct me on what is a healthy and balanced diet for me ... the exercise I take strengthens my muscles ... and replenishes my tissues ... I breathe freely and easily ... the life-giving air fills my whole body with positive energy ... as I breathe out all the negativity is expired ... I am constantly putting good things into my body ... all the exercise I take and all the food that I eat is of the right amount ... it is exactly what I need to act in a whole and dynamic way.

And as I feed my body well ... I feed my mind well ... I feed my mind with positive ... uplifting thoughts ... all the beautiful ideas that I have ... all the wonderful thoughts inspire my body to take care of itself even more ... thereby creating constant positive feedback ... which creates a glorious flowering of my mind ... and invigorating and robust health in my body ... working together ... I create this for myself.'

SCRIPTS ESPECIALLY FOR MEN

Impotence (1)

'Everybody wants to enjoy a healthy sex life ... but sometimes the desire to enjoy can get in the way of the enjoyment itself ... impotence is almost always a mental disconnection from the pleasure currently being experienced ... making love is like a roller-coaster ride ... the moment you start to think about your desire for the ride to finish is the moment that you cut off from the pleasure that you could be having ... you can even make it no fun at all!

Making love is about enjoying intimacy ... not about ending with a climax ... there is absolutely no need to perform ... nobody is judging you ... and the moment you stop worrying or analysing ... how you think you're doing ... is when you'll set yourself free ... free to really enjoy the roller-coaster ride ... the less you rush ... the more time you spend in intimacy ... the greater the trust between you and your partner ... the greater the trust ... the less you'll feel the need to perform ... at its own pace, everything will just happen naturally ... you can only truly show your love for someone else ... if they can see that you already love yourself ... this is the key ... you are their equal ... no more ... no less ... the more you love yourself ... the more they will feel your love.

Keep fit ... enjoy the exercise ... pamper yourself ... take time to really enjoy simple things ... this inner happiness is the source of the passion that you will share and enjoy with your partner ... the passion is fired but the fact that you blend with your partner is so special ... love is very special ... and so are you ... the

*longer you take enjoying your love ... the more you
release your stress ... the fitter you get ... and you'll
have a longer ... healthier life ... now you are free to
savour ... every moment ... and really enjoy your life ...
it's not a challenge ... it's a celebration.'*

Impotence (2)

'*All of us experience changes in our lives that affect us in
some way ... some changes are more subtle than others ...
sometimes they become things that we have a tendency
to focus on ... by focusing on them they seem even more
important ... we expand them out of all proportion to
their real importance ... impotence is curable ... impotence is only a temporary state for most people.*

*There are several factors that help a man to attain an
erection ... one is having a good blood circulation ... to
help your blood circulation, regular exercise is very
helpful ... especially exercising the muscle between your
legs behind the scrotum ... where the blood flow is
compressed ... helping to engorge the penis ... you can
regularly exercise this muscle by pretending to hold
back your water ... when you go to the toilet you can
stop the flow using this muscle ... this muscle is the
muscle that you need to exercise about 25 times a day,
every day ... within a very short space of time the
strengthening of this muscle will help you.*

*Other things that will improve your circulation ...
are to quit smoking and to cut down on excessive levels
of alcohol consumption ... cutting down your alcohol
consumption helps to improve the link between your
desire ... and that part of your anatomy that you need
to perform with ... to some extent, impotence is*

nothing more than a temporary disconnection of your desire from the sexual regions ... stress is a big factor in preventing us from truly experiencing our desires ... when we have other things on our mind ... we never truly enjoy what we are experiencing.

There is no need to perform and there are no rules ... just take your time and savour every moment that you spend with your partner ... the more you relax the better you feel ... whatever the state of your erection ... it's fine ... it's exactly what your body is trying to do ... the more you involve yourself in your enjoyment ... without trying to analyse your performance ... the more naturally your erection will come up ... the more you think about it ... the more difficulty you will experience ... so to free yourself from the responsibility of maintaining your erection ... is in fact to allow your body to do it naturally ... it doesn't need you to tell it to do something it has done all its life ... it just needs you to stop worrying about it ... it really is a case of when you stop worrying you have no worries ... so stop worrying about the state of your erection ... instead marvel at its ability to grow ... marvel at the amazing sensations that you can feel ... and you now for the first time really take time to explore every single part of your body around that region ... sometimes you can find erogenous areas in places you didn't expect ... and those are the places you can encourage your partner to experience for your mutual pleasure.'

Premature Ejaculation

'It is because you wish to improve your love life ... that you are now being completely honest with yourself ... you wish to increase the time you spend

making love ... but you are not doing this to just please your partner ... you are doing this to please yourself ... you wish to enjoy your love-making more ... there is no stigma involved in not being a perfect lover ... it's something that we all learn with time and that we all learn by being gentle with ourselves ... we are the worst judges of our own performance ... when we are overly self-critical we set ourselves impossible stresses that make it very hard to perform naturally ... from now on you know that your body knows exactly what to do.

From now on when you are making love ... your mind plays no part and all you need to do is listen to your body ... to feel what your body is asking you to do ... when you need to slow down ... allow yourself to slow down ... you're even allowed to withdraw completely ... there are no rules ... you do what your body wants you to do... you're allowed to stop, kiss, cuddle, caress, talk ... and when you want to start again ... you do not need to go all the way to ejaculation ... and you choose to extend the time that you take by breaking away ... or slowing down ... or taking a stop ... there are no rules ... you can even have a cup of tea ... the most important thing that you know is that ... for you ... from now on ... your love-making is something that you really enjoy ... it's something that is so natural ... there is no thought involved ... it is a complete stress-free environment ... just enjoy it ... your body ... every time it's like a holiday ... welcome to great sex.'

To Care for a Woman

'I find great pleasure in complimenting a woman ...
allowing a woman to feel good about herself because of
my sincere compliments ... and true appreciation of her
just being a woman ... whenever I am in a bar ... in a
restaurant ... or anywhere in the presence of a woman
... I am what she wants ... I enjoy the feeling of being
wanted ... and liked ... I know I am always in control ...
when I am with a woman ... no longer do I find I stut-
ter ... or am at a loss for words ... in fact, I find it easy
to talk and entertain her ... I find it easy to discover her
personality ... and establish a rapport ... quickly and
easily ... each day I feel more relaxed at the thought of
being with a woman ... all the old fears and doubts are
in the past ... no longer hindering my relationships ... as
each day goes by, I realize I feel more comfortable in
the company of a woman or women ... I have a greater
patience and a better understanding ... and will
continue to do so ... I can now make jokes with total
confidence ... with total ease ... if and when I wish to ...
have a good laugh and enjoy the woman's company ...
because I know I am no longer desperate for the
company of a woman ... as time goes by, this positive,
powerful energy that I have established allows me to
feel sensual ... calm, sexy and relaxed ... confident and
assured ... exciting ... always at the right time ... my
timing is perfect and I enjoy reading a woman ... knowing when she is really attracted to me ... being able to
give out a wanted invitation ... I learn very quickly how
to accept an invitation for romance ... just as I learn
very quickly how to give out an invitation ... an invitation that shows I am interested without intruding ...

a look or a warm smile can show my intentions.

When I feel a passion for a woman ... one whom I would really like to be with ... I easily establish a rapport ... I listen to what she is saying ... I enjoy her company ... and my inner mind creates a strategy to build a communication with her ... I programme my inner self to be caring and thoughtful ... and add the qualities that I know a woman would appreciate ... I become that person ... the person I wish to be ... to enjoy a wonderful and loving relationship ... I know that creating these natural qualities in my personality will attract the right people to me ... women who are exciting ... interesting ... bubbly ... fun to be with ... women who are faithful ... trustworthy ... caring.

I find I meet the type of woman I wish to meet ... as I am always in the right place at the right time ... I know that I am wanted by women ... just as I know that by sending out the right energy ... I will bring into my life the woman I want ... I am far more careful whom I choose for a relationship ... as I respect myself ... I want what is best for me ... and what is best for her ... I soon develop a feeling that warns me who would be hurtful for me and who would be wonderful for me ... I no longer find it difficult to take time to find the right woman ... she is worth waiting for ... my hang-ups are disappearing and I know that if I say goodbye to someone I will meet someone interesting again ... I am more aware that I don't want to become egotistical with whoever I am with ... if I'm not interested in someone I say no ... and if they are not interested in me ... I have no problem in accepting this ... as I know there is someone who is just right for me ... who is ready to come into my life.'

ESPECIALLY FOR WOMEN

The suggestions below are for changing some habits or behaviour patterns that may not be acceptable to your partner, causing rifts and distress, and which you can easily change if you wish to.

Timing for Orgasm

'You now look forward to making love to your partner ... knowing that you can enjoy a harmony that you once only dreamed of experiencing ... when you begin to make love, a wonderful dreamy relaxation comes over you ... and as you touch each other, tremendous feelings of excitement and love wash through your body ... your body becomes ready for love-making ... your nipples become hard ... and you become moist around your vagina ... to show your lover that you are ready for him ... proving he is wanted ... you have experienced masturbation and know what a climax feels like ... it is so easy now ... so easy for your inner mind ... your subconscious ... to arrange the timing of your love-making ... timing it perfectly so that you can climax with your lover ... you notice the subtle signs now so easily ... the same climax you experience on your own can now be timed to correspond with your lover's climax ... it is now so easy to do this ... you look forward to experimenting with your lover ... enjoying catering for his needs ... as well as your own ... you find you are more interested in your lover ... his body is a wonderful proof of the ingeniousness of life and the wonder of creation ... because you are so loving ...

your lover responds easily and naturally ... your inner minds working together ... and your own inner mind creates wonderful strategies ... so the timing of both of you is perfect ... in harmony with each other ... allowing you to experience a wonderful ... exciting ... and loving ... relationship.

This glorious union begins to correct other, old, incorrect programmes ... programmes that only encourage negative feelings ... hurt ... spite ... jealousy ... fear ... are no longer valid ... because you are able to fill the gaps that were otherwise left ... allowing negativity to creep in ... no more ... the result is a wonderful relationship and happiness ... kindness and caring are natural and part of your relationship ... day by day your strategies for love become more tuned in to your lover ... resulting in a fantastic union ... allowing you to feel a wonderful completeness ... success and achievement ... and deep love.'

Female Frigidity

'You are a beautiful woman ... you radiate love and glow with the knowledge that you are an absolute woman, inside and out ... you know what it feels like to be desirable and wanted ... yes, it feels so bloomingly wonderful ... that every fibre of your being is instantly switched on ... becoming alive ... soon you begin to experience the gorgeous warm sensations ... like the kiss of the lazy ... warm ... afternoon sun on your skin ... spreading all over you ... starting from the pit of your stomach ... and travelling from one cell to another ... from one nerve to another ... it is a delicious sensation ... a luxurious sensation that you allow yourself to indulge

in ... for it feels so good ... so right ... so natural.

The seed of desire is now planted in you ... this seed is now growing inside you ... as it gets bigger ... and bigger ... you let go of all your inhibitions ... you surrender to the pleasure of your senses ... every touch ... every caress ... every whisper ... carries you further into the realm of ecstasy ... the intensity gathers in momentum with every breath you take ... this is a moment of giving ... and union ... in body ... mind ... and soul ... this coming together serves to bring you and your partner ever closer ... creating a bond of understanding ... and absolute trust in each other ... it is a special time to share and enjoy.'

Nymphomania

This is a similar situation being over-sexed, as given earlier. Nymphomania is a medical dysfunction that can be dealt with by hypnosis.

'All your personal hidden reasons, which are preventing you from finding satisfaction with one man ... are no longer serving any useful purpose ... whatever still remains of these feelings is rejected by your subconscious mind ... and you are free to enjoy a full and active life with one loving partner ... who will satisfy your needs ... day by day you allow yourself to feel more alive ... more energetic and more at ease with yourself ... allow yourself to believe in a perfect special loving relationship ... imagine yourself as part of that special relationship ... confident ... loving ... perfectly satisfied with your partner in every way.

The nature of your sexuality changes as your

confidence grows ... you no longer allow sex to dominate your life ... instead you are in control of your new powerful sexuality ... which is strong ... confident ... and needs no reassurance ... you begin to attract different sorts of people and your subconscious mind guides you towards making the right choice for you... the role of sex in your life changes ... and it takes its rightful place as an integral part of a close mutually satisfying monogamous relationship.

During any periods of being alone without a partner ... you remain confident and understand that celibacy does not diminish your sexuality... you know that your sexuality is too precious to waste on meaningless affairs ... and you therefore choose your next partner with care.

Your relationships are strong ... satisfying and give you a greater feeling of self-esteem ... safety and happiness ... than you ever thought possible.'

For Larger Breasts

'In your mind's eye ... I want you to visualize a computer screen ... a large computer screen ... about 3 feet (1 metre) high ... imagine that you can see yourself full length on the screen ... you are looking at the image and considering the improvements you would like to make to your breasts ... this computer has a special drawing aid that allows you to redraw the shape of your breasts ... you test changing the shape by using the special plastic pencil provided ... you now become serious and shape your breasts to the size you would like ... you look at the rest of your body on the screen and make sure that your breasts are in proportion to what

you want ... take a moment to do this ... [60 seconds pause] ... you fix this image in your mind and each morning when you wake ... and at night before you go to sleep ... for the next three weeks you bring the image of the computer screen to your mind's eye and reshape your breasts until you are satisfied ... then you switch the screen off, knowing that your subconscious ... your inner mind ... will be working on that picture while you are getting on with your day.

Now I want you to picture yourself taking a trip into your body ... concentrate on sending an extra supply of blood to the arteries and veins in your breasts ... allowing them to feel warmer as the blood supply flows at the requited strength ... to work at increasing your breasts ... as you do this, your subconscious ... your inner mind ... starts to make your breasts firmer ... imposing their shape ... the extra energy helps your metabolism to speed up sufficiently ... so that your food intake is distributed correctly ... and you become more healthy ... and fitter than you have ever felt before ... you feel like eating healthier food ... and as you do ... your waist becomes smaller and firmer ... your whole body feels and looks better as you eat better ... and as you do this you begin to feel more like exercising ... safe, easy exercises that are food for you ... and firm up your body ... day by day, you feel fitter and fitter ... and your breasts feel firm and comfortable ... you notice they begin to take on a better shape and appearance ... and you begin to enjoy looking after your body ... it becomes natural and automatic to enjoy healthy food ... and keep your body fit by regular exercising.'

To Care for a Man

'Because you want to enjoy a full and happy loving and sexual partnership ... you need to find out what your man wants ... he will be loving to you ... but you want to find what is important to him, so that you can share your love and fulfilment with him ... this is so simple to do ... you listen to the signs ... and he will give you plenty ... signs that you have not noticed before will now become so clear ... your art of listening increases and you notice his body language ... you are so attuned to his body language that your timing is superb ... you enjoy the achievement of being his very best lover ... you work at it with ease and it's not difficult ... it's fun ... and like anything in life that's really worthwhile ... it takes some time ... effort ... and work ... to get it just right.

The work is pleasurable because you find it entertaining ... because you want to be the best lover he has ever experienced or ever will ... your inner mind finds interesting strategies to attain this ... it may mean compromise ... to entice him to want to compromise ... so he can see new and interesting ways to attain the same satisfaction and more ... as he did in the past ... but with new and inviting ways ... you realize that his body is an extension of his mind and being ... and that it is all connected ... you love his mind and you love his body ... you find that you love exploring his body ... caressing it ... loving it ... taking time with it ... the more time you spend the more it excites you ... the power of your love ... you see it as the wonderful creation that it is ... a wonderful exciting being ... that can be your special ... and private ... intimate love.'

CHAPTER
FOUR

Sexercise and Aphrodisiacs

The last two chapters have focused on showing you various ways to use your mind to help you become the person you wish to be. It is also important to look at other areas, helping you to balance your thinking and keep your mind healthy. Diet, exercise and romantic preparation should also be considered to add the finishing touches to your new lifestyle.

You may find that some of the techniques in this book seem far-fetched. Don't worry – they are presented here because they have a satisfactory success rate.

It may help to stretch your mind to realize how advanced our new knowledge is. One recent discovery, for example, is that a missing gene in mice may be linked to violent rapists. The research which has uncovered this possibility has been done at the Johns Hopkins University in Baltimore by Dr Solomon Snyder, who noticed that some brain-damaged mice went berserk. 'Their behaviour change was totally unprecedented. Even though the female mice would scream – and could even finally die from exhaustion – the males would still keep mounting them,' he says. These mutant mice were fast and fearless and six times more likely to kill than normal male mice.

All these mice were missing a brain gene that produces

nitric oxide, which in healthy male mice puts the brakes on aggressive behaviour. When the gene was chemically added, the affected mice quietened down. Dr Snyder explains that a missing gene could be the biological reason for sexual and aggressive behaviour in humans. 'What we might have here is an example of serious criminal behaviour that can be explained by a single gene defect.' Scientists now need to prove if there is a link. This would mean that all our behaviour faults could be rectified with a balancing of the chemicals in the brain. So, it surely shows the possibility of making quick, easy changes when the balance is relatively correct. And it is possible to stimulate a change in chemicals by hypnosis.

The mind can produce any disease or illness known to mankind and it can also eliminate it. That is the proven power of the mind. We have our own biochemist in our heads. The knack is to get it to work.

Meantime there are so many variables in what people want out of sex, from being taken away from it all to be pampered to being the carer of another.

Some women when they reach 50 seem to attract young men in their twenties. The tabloid press calls it the 'toy boy' syndrome. Men can also feel this strong attraction at some stage in their early manhood, should the circumstances arise. This is something that I have noticed throughout my life, this sexual electricity between the older woman and the young stud. The woman may never have fancied such a young man before, thinking him immature, but this attraction has nothing to do with mental stimulation. It seems to be *biological*. Could it be that it is nature's way of allowing us to reproduce, now we are generally living longer and women can have children to a later age? The young man is very eager to have rampant sex very often, which is very satisfying for women who have had to put up with older men becoming less active in bed. I have heard plenty of favourable reports from older women about this type of relationship, although it is generally short lived. Surprisingly, it's usually the woman who seems to get fed up first.

This arrangement is not new. In many primitive tribes an older woman was selected to train the young men of the village in the art of pleasing a woman. She would show them how to make love, acting as a sexual surrogate.

On the other hand, it is said women often lose interest in sex in their mid-forties. Where true, I have found this to be mainly through boredom with their partner. If the woman separates from the partner, her sexual appetite often resumes – if the circumstances arise and the right new partner comes along.

Then there are the incredible antics that some people perform just to stimulate a climax. My former husband, John Austin, had his own US radio show, as well as reporting from Hollywood. One of his guests was a lady sexual surrogate who participated in the clients' sexual activities, showing them where they were going wrong and actually having sex with them to help them with techniques. She had such an extraordinary story that John wrote the book already mentioned, *Sexual Surrogate*. It described the things that people get up to in order to achieve an orgasm.

One of the men could only get sexual satisfaction by believing himself to be pregnant! Of course, a man can't get pregnant, so he improvised. He would give himself an enema while lying on his stomach, filling himself full of water so he could achieve a sensation of being pregnant.

Another man could only have an orgasm by looking at buttons. It transpired that he had been dressed as a girl when he was three years old and sexually abused. His grandmother would touch him gently, turning him on. She played games with sexual connotations, using the buttons on the dresses she made him wear. He later became turned on by seeing buttons but didn't realize why – the 'why' part had been deposited in the basement of his memory filing system.

Meantime a famous sex therapist of the 1960s livened up a weary sexual relationship by getting the woman to pull her husband around the room by a string attached to his penis. They said it helped!

A prostitute explained that one of her clients got off on humiliation. He was an elderly judge, believe it or not, and he would ask her to put layers of clothes on and then strip off in front of him in a mirrored bathroom whilst he relieved himself. She told me she would much rather have had intercourse than this, as she felt very humiliated – which, of course, was his intention. She remembers walking up and down the bathroom, thinking, 'What the hell am I doing this for?' However, the client paid her well!

Much worse things go on and, unfortunately, this reflects how seriously wrong some human beings can go, forming lewd sexual habits. They become like barnacles to the abnormal sexual act – stuck with it, generally not wanting to change.

Sometimes, as with the buttons case, this is due to the inner mind locking things away. Music or an odour can activate the emotions, while the actual memory still stays suppressed. Personally, I find I can cry or get excited without knowing why. I can listen to certain types of music and feel an emotion that is so strong but I can't recall the experience that created the feeling. The memories of my six years of amnesia are lost – only occasionally snippets surface. Sadness or great joy is often the only hint. Because of my amnesia, sometimes a certain song can conjure up an emotion with such a strong sexual excitement that it reminds me of the famous scene from the movie *When Harry Met Sally*, where Meg Ryan simulated a loud orgasm in a restaurant whilst sitting opposite a man friend. Everyone in the restaurant looked on, shocked. When she had finished she continued eating her food. A woman looked at the waitress and said, 'I'll have what she's having!' That's how powerful emotions can be when out of context.

I remember meeting up with a boyfriend I hadn't seen for 17 years. I had no idea that we had had such a fantastic sexual relationship until we kissed on the station and it all come back like a tidal wave of emotion. It was like one of those kisses you see on films. After the absolute shock of finding this feeling intact, I wondered why we had ever parted. It didn't take long before it became apparent. He wanted a wife to share his life in Scotland, but I wasn't that person. Some things don't change.

While some men and women indulge in the fantasy of making love with an attractive favourite film star or other sex symbol while having intercourse with their partner, others avoid it, even though it may make the sex better. One reason for this is possibly because they are experiencing guilt feelings towards their spouses for doing so. But, through trance, an inner-self guide can be conjured up – in fact, an adult playmate – which can be extremely versatile and programmed to delight, giving another option to an otherwise uninteresting, run-of-the-mill, get-it-out-of-the-way, sexual duty *(see the adult playmate suggestion in the previous chapter, pp.71–2)*.

Traumas in a relationship can programme you for disaster. A negative relationship trigger can create an undesirable response, sometimes so severe that it can end a relationship, especially when a couple are going through a rough patch, perhaps due to outside occurrences like unemployment, which may be affecting their incomes. If one partner repeatedly hugs the other for encouragement while they are already upset – in fact in trauma from the effects of the lack of the fundamentals of life – then it is possible that when things get better this simple hug, which at one time may have helped, just becomes a trigger to bring on bad memories. The partner who once responded positively may later flinch when being approached for a hug, not consciously knowing why. But it has began to work like a trigger to a negative emotion, a reminder to the person of traumatic feelings. Not knowing the reason why they feel this way and, even worse, mistakenly thinking it is the beginning of the end of their feelings towards their partner could have serious lasting effects and damage a relationship which could have been saved with the extra knowledge of how the mind works.

If you find this may be happening to you, you can counteract it with a simple remark in your chosen suggestion, for example: *'Every time your lover or spouse hugs you you feel that wonderful love and caring which seems to just glow through your whole being, relaxing you and reminding you how special you are.'*

Knowing that this reprogramming is possible can help you and your partner to become more aware of the signs of the start of growing apart. But knowing isn't enough in itself. Hypnotherapy is able to create immediate change. It's the only therapy that can achieve this and you can use it on yourself. Just a simple suggestion in hypnosis can secure a responsibility and awareness that the hugging, or sympathy, is not just saved for traumatic experiences but is also used as a sign of love when things are happy and comfortable, a good balance of support in happy and sad times.

You may think that this is inappropriate for you. If so, just imagine how a person responds to a bad experience such as rape. They may have been well adjusted before, but now flinch at sexual involvement. A sexual action, even something as simple as a kiss, has become a reminder of a bad and humiliating experience.

LOVE HINTS

Sexual lies and charades that lead to unsatisfactory sex can be adjusted by hypnosis. The first step is to acknowledge them. You can be so wrong without realizing it.

What you may think turns someone on may, in fact, turn them off and, what is worse, this could have been a secret lie that has been going on for years! A woman may believe that her man likes her in black stocking tops, for instance, the modern version that stay up by themselves, when he has only pretended to do so and he actually likes the old-fashioned suspender belts. She is just presuming they are the same. Or he may think there is no need to bring her gifts or buy her flowers because she once said she didn't need them when they first met. People change, want change and it is important to change with them.

I have been on the other side of therapy for so long. I worked as a consultant hypnotherapist to a romantic hotel on Langkawi Island in Malaysia, which is so exotic it specializes in honeymoon couples. So many times I talked to a beautiful couple at the cocktail bar or in the pool – couples who were holding hands, kissing and saying how much in love they were. But when one – or sometimes both – came to have therapy, say for stopping smoking or a phobia, the story was often very different. Little irritations came out in hypnosis that were more than likely going to develop into a problem if not dealt with. A relationship can be so much more successful if these areas are straightened out at the beginning. The simple blueprint plan in Chapter 3 can help instruct the subconscious and bring about a greater compatibility *(see pp.58–65)*.

It is well worth doing your homework on finding out what your partner's likes are, not just sexually but in other areas. Your lover might just be being polite when you ask them if they like the same things as you do and they agree. They might just be trying to please you. Haven't you ever noticed that you seem to develop a taste for a certain type of music when you fancy someone and then you go back to your own tastes after the relationship is over? Find out what your partner's favourite music is for making love. They may not like music at all, but certain music does create a mood and can stimulate sexual feelings even more. I happen to like Donna Summer but someone else may prefer Bach or, indeed, brass bands. You need to compromise but in a sharing capacity.

Why not plan a special night or weekend? Make it extraordinary, different. Music, decor and lighting are all part of the trappings of a wonderful night of passion. Don't be so egotistical as to presume that because sex is great now you can drop the frills. For instance, if you decide to give your loved one a massage, ensure your hands are warm, make sure the room is at the right temperature and allow yourself plenty of time to enjoy each other. There's no rush.

Make sure your loving place is clean and tidy. Flowers or fragrances, incense or oils are important, helping stroke the senses. Massage is wonderful. It is very easy to learn and can be so rewarding. Take a bath or shower together, washing away the cares of the day. Use an induction tape – it acts like a massage. You can design one specially for relaxing and maybe put some mood music behind it. This is very easy to do on a decent tape recorder.

When you have relaxed and changed the mood of a busy day to the luxury of indulging in each other. Stay in the present and don't just fantasize. Immediately, fantasizing disassociates you from the 'now'. Remember the difference between thinking about eating an ice cream and actually eating one? So be together, in the 'now'. Eye contact is very important, too. It will keep you in tune with your partner. Let your body do what it wants to do and enjoy it!

Love List

When you fall in love with someone, you don't look for the faults. When you fall out of love they stand out like neon lighting. The following list helps you to acknowledge your and your partner's faults in the early stages and therefore allows you to create strategies to compensate.

1 Clean up your act by spring cleaning your mind or you will attract someone with as much negative baggage as yourself *(see blueprint in Chapter 3, pp.58–65)*.
2 Remember that a person can make you feel loved and nurtured because they know how to do it. They don't necessarily have to love you. The problem is your instincts will not automatically come to your rescue. Quite simply, you are open to being conned.
3 Keep certain parts of your mind free for your own space. Don't give it all away or your partner will have nothing left to want and then the boredom will set in.
4 Work at your relationship. You can do this by respecting yourself and your lover. If you lose respect for yourself and get slovenly, then your lover may also change, perhaps moving away from you. In fact, you will be more or less throwing the towel in, leaving it to fate to break things up, when the saboteur is actually you.

APHRODISIACS

*('Any food, drug, etc., that stimulates
the sexual appetite')*

Money, food and belief are all aphrodisiacs. Belief works, even if it is totally unfounded. I am preparing to open a stress release clinic in the South Pacific in the Kingdom of Tonga. The Prime Minister has just given me two acres on his beach-front land opposite a phenomenon called the 'blowholes'. These are natural water fountains, shooting up from the sea hundreds of feet into the air. (Now I have the land I will be expecting investment – creative visualization at its best!) I was also given the honour of planting a tree in Tonga and discussed aphrodisiacs with the Director of Agriculture. Tonga grows vanilla for export and he explained that it has to be fertilized by hand, which is a very sensitive and delicate job. In order for him to get the best out of his workers, in terms of both speed and sensitivity, he told them that the plant was an aphrodisiac. The workers became very happy at their work, even though the truth was questionable!

My first introduction to aphrodisiacs was in the 1980s when I interviewed author Diane Warburton, who had just published a book called *The A–Z of Aphrodisiacs* (Quartet, 1987). Money was top of the list, but I learned that healthy eating is a good runner-up. There are certain foods that serve as incentives for both yourself and your lover.

Spanish fly and oysters are two of these, but it soon became apparent that there was more to aphrodisiacs than this. It was such a fascinating subject that I decided to orga-nize a celebrity panel to sample a 'menu for love' for a magazine I was launching. This was in the champagne '80s and money was being spent freely. The venue was the

Hippodrome, at the time owned by Peter Stringfellow, and I used the occasion as an excuse for a very small, select launch party for my magazine. Selecting the panel was fun and I ended up with eight very interesting and knowledgeable celebrities who knew how to enjoy themselves. Among them were Cynthia Payne, actress Sally Thomsett and Sam Connery, the then Levi jeans heart-throb.

Diane Warburton loved the idea of an aphrodisiac party and, along with Nicholas, head chef at Stringfellow's, devised a marvellous and scrumptious aphrodisiac menu including such wonders as truffles. Very expensive, the menu was also dynamic, with some very interesting results. I found out later that one of the female guests had met a man and checked into a hotel that evening, even though one-night stands were definitely not her normal behaviour.

Diane explained that it is important to know how aphrodisiacs work. They can act as a diuretic, a laxative or a stimulant for a particular area. They do not work instantly, rather like, for example, an aspirin which needs half an hour to take effect. Thus, people who complain that an aphrodisiac is not working are probably not allowing the necessary time.

An important factor is that you must not eat too much because an overloaded stomach is definitely not conducive to love-making. A perfect starter would be snails' eggs on lightly buttered toast, for example. Eating a light meal is good, perhaps not in the evening but some time during the day, and you must be rested.

Nicholas created the menus below. He told me that when preparing an aphrodisiac menu for a TV programme, he read a few books and came to the conclusion that 90 per cent of all foods were supposed to have aphrodisiac qualities! Certainly, shellfish, asparagus and wild mushrooms were well up most lists. But potatoes were one of the few foods that definitely were not classed in any sexual category. I think it's a matter of individual taste. What might be an aphrodisiac to one person could be a passion-killer to another.

SUGGESTED MENUS FOR LOVE

*Whitstable oysters served on ice with snails' eggs
and beluga caviar*

*Asparagus garnished with fresh tomato and glazed
with hollandaise sauce*

*A combination of chicken, mussels and black truffles
lightly steamed and presented on a warm vinaigrette*

*A selection of tender vegetables sautéd in butter with
new potatoes*

Pickled peaches, honey, Royal Jelly, truffles, sugared almonds and champagne could also be included in a hamper of passion.

SEXERCISES

Exercise for both men and women is very important to a good sexual relationship. Vaginal exercises for the woman entail simply squeezing your vaginal muscles together. Scrotum exercises for the man are well worth the effort. For both sexes the exercises take less than a minute but can make all the difference to responses and love-making. Other exercises meanwhile help to firm up important areas.

The abbreviation s.o.a. stands for sex organ area.

Scrotum Exercise

There are several factors that help a man to attain an erection. It is important to have good blood circulation. This can be improved by regular exercise, especially exercising the muscle between your legs behind the scrotum. This is where the blood flow is compressed, helping to engorge the penis. You can regularly exercise this muscle by pretending to hold back your water. When you go to the toilet you can stop the flow by using this muscle. You need to exercise this muscle about 25 times a day, every day, and within a very short space of time the strengthening of this muscle will help you in your love-making *(see also pp.115–16)*.

Vaginal Exercise

This is very similar to the scrotum exercise. You tense the bunch of muscles in the way you would if you were trying to stop yourself from urinating and hold them for 5 seconds, 15 times a day, and then let go. This exercise will firm the muscles up, instead of them sagging with age, and you will find you have more control in the sexual regions. This is a very good exercise to begin if you are over 40.

Here are some other physical exercises that will tone up those sexual muscles...

For Women

Stand erect with your feet apart. Squat about halfway down, hands behind your neck. Thrust your s.o.a. downward and backward as far as it will go and hold for 6 seconds.

Sit on the floor, legs straight and slightly apart, hands on the floor behind your buttocks. Thrust your s.o.a. upward and forward as high as it will go and hold for a count of 10.

Sit on the floor, legs straight and slightly apart, hands on the floor behind your buttocks. Thrust your s.o.a. downwards and backwards as far as it will go and hold for 6 seconds.

Lie back on the floor with your knees bent and feet slightly apart. Thrust your s.o.a. downwards as far as it will go and hold for 6 seconds.

Lie face down on the floor with your legs straight and slightly apart. Bend your elbows, and place your forearms and the palms of your hands on the floor beneath your chest. Raise your upper body so that your chest does not touch the floor. Thrust your s.o.a. forward and upward as high as it will go and hold.

Lie face down on the floor as instructed immediately above. With weight of your upper body resting on your forearms, thrust your s.o.a. downward and backward as far as it will go and hold.

Stand erect with your feet spread apart. Thrust your hips strongly to the left and hold for 6 seconds. Relax. Thrust your hips strongly to the right and hold for 6 seconds.

Lie flat on your back with your legs straight and slightly apart. Squeeze your buttocks tightly together and hold for 6 seconds.

Lie face down on the floor. Bend your elbows and place your forearms on the floor beneath your chest. Raise your upper body so that your chest does not touch the floor. Squeeze your buttocks tightly together and hold for 6 seconds.

Lie with your back on the floor, knees slightly bent and together, arms beside your head. Squeeze your legs together as hard as you can while you count to 10.

Lie face down on the floor, arms in front of your body and legs together. Squeeze your legs together as hard as you can while you count to 10.

Sit on the edge of a chair. Place a ball between your knees and squeeze your legs together as hard as you can while you count to 10 for approximately 6 seconds.

Lie down on the floor, knees slightly bent and together, arms beside your head. Squeeze your legs together as hard as you can for 6 seconds.

For Men

Stand erect with your feet slightly apart, hands on thighs. Pull in your stomach and thrust your s.o.a. forward and upward as high as it can go. Hold this position for a count of 10 and then relax.

Stand erect with your feet slightly apart and hands on hips. Lift your buttocks up as you hollow your back and thrust your s.o.a. downwards and backwards as far as it will go. Hold this position for a count of 10.

Get down on your hands and knees on the floor. Spread

your knees slightly. Thrust your s.o.a. forward and upward as high as it will go and hold for 6 seconds.

Stay on your hands and knees. Spread your knees slightly. Thrust your s.o.a. downward and backward as far as it will go and hold.

Lie flat on your back with your legs straight and spread slightly apart, arms alongside your body, palms on the floor. Arch your body as strongly as you can, thrusting your s.o.a. up as high as possible and hold for a count of 10.

Lie flat on your back with your knees slightly bent and your feet on the floor. Tense your abdominal muscles as hard as you can and hold for 10 counts. Relax. Stretch your legs out and roll over onto your left side. Tense your abdominal muscles as hard as you can and hold for 10 seconds. Roll over onto your right side and repeat.

Lie flat on your back, hands on your thighs. Raise your head and shoulders off the floor, and slide your hands up your knees so you are curled forward. Hold this position for 10 counts.

Lie face down on the floor, legs straight and together, with your hands clasped behind your head. Raise your chest and legs off the floor by arching your back as strongly as possible. Hold this position for 6 seconds.

FIVE

*'I have one redeeming feature:
I am a learner, not a know-it-all'*
JOHN

I have chosen the following case histories in order to give you an idea of how deeply rooted some problems can be when, on the surface, they look fairly ordinary – or vice versa.

Much of my research for this book was tailored towards helping you to find and attract Ms or Mr Right. The material gave me fascinating case histories, some almost beyond belief. The changes that were seen after simple suggestion hypnosis were exciting, giving a better understanding of how the mind works in romantic relationships.

The case histories illustrate how sophisticated the human mind is and how many sexual problems and dilemmas can be traced back to long-forgotten traumas that defy conscious logic. So these examples will add to your overall knowledge and help you to identify more clearly your own problems and to understand them better. I have changed the names of the subjects to protect their identity.

ELIZABETH

Her own words before the treatment:

I am single, 55 years old, youthfully attractive. I have never been married. In the last few years there's been nobody special but lots of boyfriends who were wrong for me. I don't really understand it. I am attractive, accomplished, talented and have a lovely home, and yet I am alone.

The women in my family – my mother, aunts, etc. – always attached a lot of importance to looking good and having good taste. I thought that was what was required to have a man in my life. I've been amazed when I have seen really plain women with gorgeous men.

My parents separated when I was 16, although they had never really been together since I was five. I never saw my mother and father embrace or be loving towards each other. But, then, my father was hardly ever around, always working abroad, so I and my two brothers were brought up by my mother. We had a very happy childhood. I think with hindsight that it was easier being with one parent. But, on the other hand, I had no example of a loving relationship, no role model.

In my younger days I didn't think about marriage. I had no difficulty attracting men, but never found one I wanted to be with for very long, and they never pressured me very much.

I feel very lonely sometimes. I wonder if I'm destined to live the rest of my life alone. Recently on holiday, I had a short, sweet romance. It was so beautiful to be loved and kissed and treated with tenderness. It's been quite a few years now since I had a boyfriend. Just being kissed and held seemed like a miracle – why should this be so? I'd like a man in my life, a partner to live with and share experiences with and enjoy life together. Why should it be a rare thing for me to be held and cherished?

Just about all my friends have partners now, so my relationship with them has changed. Whereas once we were all single and did things together, now they are all in relationships and do things with their partners. Now, I have no man and I don't really have friends, either. I'd like to meet someone to share a happy life with. I don't want to be alone anymore. I want to be in a joyful loving relationship and I'd like to be married. I think a relationship is sacred.

The 'short, sweet' relationship that Elizabeth had encountered was a torrid, wonderful, exciting, love lust, registering ten on the Richter scale. She had met her love on holiday on one of her many trips abroad and had a roller-coaster experience. After spending many happy nights fantasizing about him on her return to the UK, she realized it was wrong for her, leading nowhere except to eventual hurt. One evening, just before she slept, she gave herself some self-hypnosis and made a conscious decision to end the relationship. The next morning she woke up without the feeling – it had gone, evaporated, disintegrated. All the pining and petty jealousies were gone too, and Elizabeth was left with only sweet, wonderful memories.

If I hadn't encountered this kind of feeling myself, I would not have believed it possible. I would have put my own experience down to my erratic memory. It started with my talking to a girlfriend who has had a wonderful, full life. Used to mingling with the rich and famous, she even had a boyfriend who sent a tanker of oil to her door because she had run out of fuel for her central heating during a shortage. She has a picture of herself with Ronald Reagan on her mantelpiece but subtly changes the subject when I ask her about it. My friend said that she could just fall out of love in an instant if a guy gave her a problem. I liked that idea, because I didn't realize someone could control their emotions so well.

On my next trip to Malaysia, I fell hopelessly in love with an Asian billionaire I met at a carpet auction. I realize many will not believe me but I had already been offered a million pounds by another man to sleep with him – and turned it down! I knew it was available because I was actually shown the money in cash. It was just before the controversial film *Indecent Proposal* came out, in which Demi Moore was offered a million dollars to sleep with Robert Redford and she did, causing chaos. I had the courage to refuse – but that's probably because the guy didn't look like Robert Redford! My billionaire was different. I was crazy about him. I would have died for him. We were both single and decided to stay together – not a good idea. If you think a millionaire is hard to deal with, that's nothing to my billionaire.

I realized that I would have to drop out of my life and follow him around like a love-lost fawn. That prospect wasn't very pretty and, considering that the car accident that caused my amnesia happened after the break up of one of those ten-on-the-Richter-scale-type relationships, another impossible love wasn't very tempting. It spelt *danger*, in fact.

My billionaire also did something that I found unacceptable, not terribly important in a general sense but important to me. That did it. I made the decision to get out of the affair and, like magic, I woke up the next morning out of love. My decision, and being armed with the information from my girlfriend, made it possible for me to move out of this dangerous liaison. I would have probably blamed it on my faulty memory if Elizabeth hadn't confided in me that she, too, had made that definite decision and woken up the next morning out of love, with just sweet memories. I felt so wonderfully free and very relieved to have escaped running down the wrong road. It also confirmed my view that if you can get out of a potentially hurtful relationship with no pain, you can also get back into one that is worthwhile.

A good spring clean of the mind can definitely be a deterrent to any tendency you have to keep on attracting the wrong person. The less trauma baggage you carry, the less trauma baggage you will attract.

Elizabeth expressed her reactions after just one session with suggestion hypnosis:

> The most effective part of the session was being able to look back on my past relationships and see how they really were – certainly not ideal. It was actually funny to look back to see how I chose the wrong people, time and time again.
>
> Since I stopped doing that, I have had no relationships. I must have closed down for protection. I can now see why this strange protection has been created. I realize that I needed protection from the fellows I was attracting.
>
> I remembered I got an infection that went to my kidneys. I was incredibly ill. Then I had another fling and got some other sexually transmitted disease. I realized I was completely on the wrong path.
>
> Today I feel really different about this whole thing. I really feel the therapy has opened me up, woken up my feelings. But now I feel I will choose better men in future. I no longer feel the need to close down completely.

Hypnosis can modify this strategy of the subconscious but only if you are not going to carry on with the same behaviour. That is where the suggestions help, as new programmes, to create a modification in the mind.

JIM

One of my clients in the entertainment industry, whom I will call Jim, has always cross dressed. He did not consider it a problem himself. His second wife, however, found it difficult to deal with, as had his first wife also. The difference was, he had told his second wife about his preference before they married. She had accepted it initially – but obviously without a preview. When he actually dressed as a woman, she found it unacceptable and a real turn-off.

Although they both agreed that they loved each other, Jim's preference stood in the way of either being sexually satisfied. If this issue could be dealt with, they agreed they would have a chance of a very satisfying sexual relationship.

Although this may seem an extreme case, the same problem could come about if, say, one partner is not happy with oral sex or the other wanting to view pornographic videos. In order to find a solution it would need one, or both, to compromise.

The choice had been made in this case – the wife had at first agreed to her husband's tastes but had not followed through, thereby creating a dilemma. They had come to me for advice and to see if hypnosis could help. First, I had to establish whether they were happy with each other as a couple and then I needed to find out if there was a compromise that could be agreed on.

The wife's ideal was simple. She wanted her husband to change but she realized that she had accepted the situation before she married him and understood he did have a point when he suggested that she should try to deal with her distaste in therapy. He enjoyed the way he was and had no intention of changing. He had always been this way. In fact, he seemed rather proud of it. He was not ashamed and believed his taste for cross dressing to be no more harmful than a sex aid. 'I do not break the law, I am not a murderer or a thief and I am not gay,' was his reasoning.

Jim explained he was brought up in a female-dominated family and remembered being allowed to dress up in his mother's silk stockings when he was three, using safety pins as the suspenders. His mother neither stopped nor encouraged him. By the age of six, he achieved an erection by wearing female underwear and it progressed to his wearing women's clothes and make-up. He described the feeling of dressing as a woman as 'pure heaven' and felt he had been cheated by not having a vagina. He explained that if he were 20 years younger he would have had a sex change and that his frustration was that he had not been born a woman – yet he did not have a desire for men. He also believed he would have liked to act out a lesbian life similar to the well-publicized story of a sailor who had surgery and underwent a sex change. It was a rather unusual story because when the sailor became a woman she had an affair and lived with another woman in a lesbian relationship.

Jim was small, balding and very hairy. Even his back was hairy, so dressing as a woman took time. He explained he could spend a 'glorious' hour shaving his legs. He never wanted, or had any intention of having, anal sex and thought it strange that men would consider this appropriate. That, in his eyes, would be the act of a homosexual – and he wasn't gay. He had been disappointed in his wife and felt cheated, as she had accepted the fact that he cross dressed before they married.

They both agreed that she should use self-hypnosis to lift her inhibitions about his preferences, so she would not be turned off by it. I explained that the subconscious would only make a change if it was what she really wanted. The treatment worked and the result was a much happier relationship all round. They both got what they wanted: the ability to make each other happy. There was no doubt they loved each other and had been happy together in every other respect – but now it was even better.

This was quite radical, but Jim's wife realized that even if he had agreed to have therapy for change, it was unlikely that it would have worked, simply because he liked being the way he was. It was his comfort zone. Alternatively, she could deal with lifting her inhibitions to allow her to enjoy a sexual relationship.

I had explained that, in a similar example, if someone came to me for therapy for stopping snoring, I would suggest that their partner would be better advised to have the therapy. The snoring would lull them into a wonderful relaxation and sleep would come very quickly and easily. In fact, the sound of their partner snoring would give them a wonderful feeling of comfort and safeness, relieving the pressures of the day.

LEON

Leon was recommended to me by my favourite psychiatrist, who used to send me extraordinary patients. Leon was one of my most memorable, because I learned so much from his case.

He had been madly in love with a girl but they had broken up well over a year before his visit. He was the son of a doctor, in his early twenties, good looking and with a lovely personality. His problem was that he couldn't get over his love affair and still had a fixation for the girl. It was so obsessive that he thought about her 90 per cent of the day. His mind went round and round with 'what ifs': *What if I had treated her better? What if I had curbed my jealousy?* And so on.

Generally, such a trauma over a broken love affair should begin to clear in about six months, when the mind has begun to adjust. Having such an obsession for so long afterwards was causing Leon to become very depressed. He was on tranquillizers to enable him to get through the days.

Leon said everything about the relationship had been fantastic, including the sex. However if I told him he was lucky to have known someone so perfect, he would contradict his last statement and go into a lengthy description of her faults. If I later mentioned even one of her faults, he would say how spectacular the relationship had been. I couldn't win with him – a sure sign of a confused mind.

He was already in another relationship but this didn't disturb his obsession. Obviously, the new relationship was a wrong choice again, due to a confused mind.

Fortunately, hypnosis was able to unscramble the mess and after five sessions he was only thinking about his previous love for about 5 per cent of the day. Their time together had become distant memories, which he requested to melt away naturally, allowing him to get on with his life.

Of course, it wasn't his relationship that was the problem at all. The real problem was, he was very screwed up and needed to get his mind unscrambled, so he could attract the right person. I saw him a few years later. He was in a happy relationship and looked a different person, calm, confident and even better looking, with a new sophisticated attitude to life.

HELEN AND JOHN AND
JANE AND TONY

In my research for this book, I decided to bring a few people together with the intention of using the blueprint therapy treatment described in Chapter 3 to help their sexual and communication relationships.

Both couples already had very satisfactory sexual relationships, marred only by a lack of communication in certain areas. These particular couples would never have normally come for therapy because they believed their sex life to be great enough as it was. However I conducted a group therapy and asked them to contact me a week later with some feedback.

The first couple, Helen and John, were in their fifties. Helen was a relaxation therapist and John a solicitor. Their attitudes towards my experiment were different. He was very sceptical but she was optimistic. She explained that John was the romantic, whereas she was very practical. He made love absolutely wonderfully – in fact, the best she had ever experienced – but not very often. It had made her wonder if it was her fault.

Helen called me a week later to report there had been a definite shift in their relationship from her side. She found she was playing romantic music, like Julio Iglesias, something she would not normally think of, and feeling very much more complete with her sexuality. She had noticed this when she went to a party during the week. She no longer felt she had to prove anything and had realized that her life was no longer run by sex. She felt clearer about her sexuality. Quite happy that sex with John was already brilliant, in addition she found that it didn't really matter that it was

infrequent because she no longer doubted herself. Her attitude had changed and she saw the positive side of having a
wonderful lover. She began to count her blessings and realize
how lucky she was to have such an erotic and caring
husband. Because of this new attitude, she was communicating more with her husband and acting and feeling more
romantic – a new emotion they could share. They hadn't
been able to share this before because she had not previously
felt romantic – it was a new experience for her.

As I was writing about Helen, John called me. He said he
owed me an apology:

> If you had asked me yesterday if there was any change,
> I would have said no. With my workload, I reserve sex
> for weekends, but this weekend I had a headache which
> would normally have prevented me from any sexual
> activity. But I found it just didn't matter. We had a
> wonderful time. I noticed Helen was more active and it
> was great. I felt young again. I just did what my body
> liked and enjoyed myself.

When I told him that a lot of couples resisted the necessity to
improve their love life because they thought it was great as it
was, his response was: 'I have one redeeming feature: I'm a
learner, not a know-it-all.'

That is probably why John makes such a wonderful lover.
However, I felt I had proved my point – that, yes, you can
make something great even better! I noticed when Helen tele-
phoned me that she was far more complimentary about
John, sounding more like he was a new lover. When John
called me, I found the same response. Both were like a pair of
honeymooners! They sounded so happy that I felt all my
research had been worth it.

Tony and Jane were much younger, in their twenties. Tony

was a creative person, a photographer, video producer and a creative designer. Jane was also very creative, but more negative in her approach to life. The therapy allowed them to communicate more, to be able to talk to each other about the problems that were hindering the relationship. They had just come back together after a trial separation. Their sex life had been very good anyway, but after the one suggestion therapy session they definitely found a difference – a greater completeness, with a new understanding and ability to get things out into the open.

Tony:

I felt I had more time. Things seemed even more natural. That is, being natural was even easier, and whilst this doesn't sound very much, it certainly was. The evening of the therapy we were both tired, and I was definitely overworked, but we enjoyed the best love-making for ages.

Jane:

The next day I felt very good. I had a new lease of energy, there was definitely an instant improvement. I made two discoveries: things had to get worse before they could get better and we had to clear some things up, so we could enjoy our relationship.

Each found it difficult to put into words, but they had both experienced a noticeable improvement in their relationship. Tony and Jane had to come to terms with a few things that had broken them up in the first place. I saw Tony quite regularly and was able to observe the change myself. He sounded more logical about how he felt and he was really acting upon what he said, rather than just letting things ride and hope for the best. It was as if everything seemed clearer to him. And, yes, it had helped their sex relationship in a very important area – real communication.

You may think your sex life can't be improved, but have you ever noticed that on the odd occasion it can be more wonderful than ever? If you can admit this, then of course it can be improved by creating more of those extra-wonderful nights.

I once watched a TV documentary on a Native American tribe, the Cherokee. It showed a group of them regularly getting together to try and maintain their culture and language, which were fast dying out. A young boy who was interviewed said that his grandmother had taught him why it was so important to keep their own language. She said that the English language was like a minute black-and-white television, while the Cherokee language was like a gigantic colour cinema screen. They had so many words to explain feelings.

The point I am making here is that we often find it difficult to relate new feelings – there doesn't seem to be the vocabulary for them. But Native Americans have experienced trance for centuries as part of their culture and so have developed a more descriptive language to allow for these many states of mind.

ALENA AND JEROLD

I was lecturing abroad when I was asked to do some therapy with a couple. I already knew Jerold, but not his wife. I had treated him for stopping smoking and then for a drink problem two years before. He had been a heavy drinker but had lost his tolerance for alcohol and it had been interfering with his lifestyle as a health trainer. He would be quite obnoxious to people when he drank, which was every night, and then he spent the next day apologizing. With a new programme in place, his life changed. You know a problem has been solved when the person who has hypnosis to give up an unwanted habit has no regrets or feelings of loss, just a great relief.

So, with his outstanding belief structure already in place, when Jerold told me he wanted to get back together with his wife so they could be more compatible and asked me if I could treat them both, I was glad to help.

It was a similar story to that of many couples who want to get back together because of their young children – but not necessarily for the right reasons. It is quite an intricate position when doing the couples therapy because the therapist has to be so careful to keep each one's secrets, whilst untangling the mess they have created.

Jerold's complaints about Alena seemed valid – with couples, they often are. Her nagging behaviour stemmed from childhood traumas and attitudes developed for protection. Her strategies worked for her but later became an irritation to Jerold.

Alena told me that Jerold didn't like her wearing make-up, so she had become sloppy. From a woman used to power dressing, she now spent most of her time in leggings and T-shirts. Her whole image had changed and she told me that some of her friends didn't recognize her any longer. When I broached this with Jerold, his story was a little different. When he had said he didn't like her wearing make-up, he meant the 'power' make-up she wore for work. To him, it was unfeminine. Alena had misinterpreted his remark and obliged by not wearing any make-up at all. She thought she was pleasing him. The result was a drastic change in her own image, which she didn't like and neither did he. There was a lack of communication, resulting in an accumulation of problems and a change of behaviour in them both whereby they simply grew more apart.

In my first therapy with couples I see them both together. The irritations soon surface. The next two to three sessions I see them separately on a one-to-one basis. Those irritations – even something that looks simple, such as nail-biting, nagging, over-dressing or under-dressing – can be the key to the trauma problems. The lover is always the first to see these faults when the relationship is in trouble. Relatives generally think these flaws are part of the personality, while the person accepts them as traits or parts of their make-up.

Once the treatment is completed, then both have a better chance of a happy relationship – but not always together. The advantage is that they will see it sooner, rather than later.

In the case of Jerold and Alena, they stayed together for a year and then separated. They had genuinely tried to make a go of it and then, realizing it finally wasn't going to work, they were able to release each other from what would have been a lifetime of suppression and falseness. Now they are living happily apart and are very good friends, their children ensuring a lasting bond between them, while at the same time they are both free to find a more compatible partner.

My own experience had taught me, after all my years of practice, that you can fall out of love in an instant. But certain things are very important in establishing compatibility in certain areas – the home and music, for instance. Music can be a wonderful thing for togetherness – especially when making love to it. If you are truly together, sharing pleasure in the same kind of music, then each partner can reach a higher level of excitement, rather than just one experiencing utopia, creating a wonderful, deeper bonding.

Even a basic area like home decoration can be an important cause of compatibility or friction. If one partner doesn't like the other's taste, they will always find it hard to settle

HYPNOSEX

and feel truly at home. The dissatisfied one becomes restless but doesn't really know why.

One of my clients reported that her husband was very uncaring and she felt used and put upon. She said that a few years earlier he had agreed to the home being redecorated, but after she had bought the wallpaper and paint he would not help at all. They had two children and she found the job hard to do by herself but she was determined and managed to finish it.

Now it was time to redecorate again. The same thing happened – he agreed, so she bought the wallpaper and paint and began stripping the walls. However, when the husband got home from work all he did was complain about the mess she had made and refused to help.

On the face of it, he sounded rather uncaring. But, as in most cases, the husband's story was a little different. He said he wouldn't help because his wife had terrible taste and he didn't see why he should help with the redecorating, especially as she had not consulted him when choosing the paper and paint. He felt frustrated and alienated. It was bad enough having to live in a home he already didn't like without helping to make it look even more monstrous, so he refused, a silent objection which she didn't understand. She loved her home with her rather gaudy taste, while he felt restless, wanting to get out and go to the pub with his mates.

Unfortunately, this couple did not return after the first session, so I am unable to tell you whether they ultimately resolved their problem. However, I have included the case history to illustrate that compromising isn't always the answer. It doesn't solve the problem of never feeling at home in your own home. Compromising can mean that neither party is settled. They may feel more at home elsewhere – and that creates the setting for possible infidelity. It's best to check out these important basics at the beginning of a

132

relationship, not after the honeymoon. It's no use just pretending you like what your partner likes because these little irritations can ultimately be the point that determines whether you stay together or not.

A BIZARRE CASE OF INCEST

I have a dear friend, also a hypnotherapist, who seems to get the most extraordinary people in for therapy. One of her case histories was remarkably similar to a storyline in the TV series *Cracker*, about a police psychiatrist. The story was about incest but with a very different angle. The main character was a female serial killer in her early twenties, good looking and in a reasonable job, who killed young men she picked up for one-night stands. The whole story had the viewer believing her father had sexually abused her, as he had her sister. The truth was that he hadn't and, because she was the only daughter who hadn't been sexually molested, she felt unloved, ugly, distrustful and a mass of emotional rage which ended up in her venting her self-hatred by killing.

The killing was only a storyline but the rest of the facts were very similar to my friend's client's case, except that the incest was far worse. Almost everyone had been with everyone else – mothers with grandfathers, grandfathers with nieces, fathers with daughters. New husbands came and went and seemed to take turns with the sisters and the mother. In fact, the abuse went back three generations. The one exception was my colleague's client, who had not been touched. Astonishingly, she suffered the most damaging lack of self-worth, because she *hadn't* been molested. Her problem was, the incest was part of her life, a normality to her. Unfortunately, she didn't finish her treatment.

My friend also had a wife who came to see her about her

husband's philanderings with other women. It turned out he had been exposed in the Sunday newspapers with a few wives in tow. They all found out and took him to court. While his wife saw my friend in her capacity as a therapist, the husband was secretly calling her to make a date, saying he was using her relaxation tapes to accompany his masturbation. My friend confronted them both together about it. The wife was extremely distraught but the situation would only change if the husband were willing to change. But, of course he wasn't. He took the view that it was his wife's problem, not his!

ANTONY

I met Antony at a sophisticated workshop. He was airing his views to the participants. He explained that he had spent the whole of the 1970s, '80s and now the '90s going to these workshops. He had been all over the world to see gurus and indulge in spiritual meditation and yet he felt extreme despair, pain and apprehension and a deep sense of loneliness the whole time. So, despite spending 25 years attending the best workshops, he still hadn't changed. He also complained about always ending up in the wrong relationship. They never worked out. I looked at him and told him bluntly that I wouldn't touch him with a barge pole! I meant it, too – all that excess baggage he was carrying would have frightened me off. I was longing for a chance to work with him, though, and offered to treat him as part of my research for the book. Below are the results.

Antony has a marvellous plummy voice and is wonderfully intelligent, with a charming sense of humour. I mention this, as I enjoy working with someone who is going to give me a run for my money. The three words that summed his ife up before hypnotherapy were 'depression', 'pain' and apprehension'. But after the third session, the words to describe his new attitude to life were 'peace', 'love' and 'joy'. This was an extraordinary change.

Let Antony tell it in his own words, after two sessions of treatment:

I approached the idea of hypnotherapy with a great deal of scepticism, having spent years in various encounter groups and self-improvement seminars. It was much to my surprise that after one session of hypnotherapy I found not only had a pain in my groin area become greatly relieved but after a few days completely disappeared. [I didn't even know he had been in such physical discomfort.]

Additionally, after the second session I found my self-confidence had become greatly improved. Without doubt, hypnotherapy has opened a way for me to fully experience being myself.

Nothing was stopping me having a relationship but I think it just brought me back to my consciousness, and what I was experiencing was that all the stuff that was going on was just a story and it wasn't me. I remembered all of the pain. I didn't remember the joy, so my editing system must have been telling me to remember rejection, not success.

The other day I was rather chuffed. I was doing some business transaction with a person with an incredible mathematical mind, the sort of high-powered guy who is very quick to get answers, yet I got the figures right and he got them wrong. I'm beginning to find myself. I would never have had the courage to do this before. Also, without much effort, I have had three journalists and one TV crew round this week. Life become a lot easier. The therapy seems to have opened the channel that sends out the energy to the universe.

After his third treatment:

Writing a testimonial always puts me on the spot, particularly when dealing with such personal matters as therapy. Having spent years examining my navel and participating in training, including EST, TM, encounter groups, 10 days' silent meditation at the feet of Tibetan Masters, hours of yoga and debating aspects of the *Bhagavad Gita*, to give a sincere answer on the value of hypnotherapy has presented me with some turmoil.

First, my comments are not based on a comparison but on the benefits four weeks after Valerie took me under her wing. I have been experiencing the fear of being 40-something and questioning all aspects of my life, including why have I never married or ever resolved my relationship with my mother and my fear that the slightest ache or bump on my body could be a life-threatening illness.

So, I entered hypnotherapy with a jaundiced eye, to which I will add the hidden agenda that as my mother, coincidentally, is a hypnotherapist, it had little appeal, other than as another trinket to add to my navel-gazing experiences.

However, I have had tremendous value from hypnotherapy in only three sessions. Aching pains in my testicles have gone, I feel comfortable at the idea of writing to my mother, with whom I have had little contact for many years, a renewed self-confidence with women, to the point of seriously thinking that a partnership could be a really nice experience, and a willingness to take a risk in my business life after spending several years sitting on the fence.

Only three sessions to change someone's life! Just because someone has suffered a trauma-related problem for 25 painful years, does not mean it needs any more lengthy therapy than a trauma that caused a fear of spiders or bridges.

When Antony went into regression, he went to a time when he was a baby. He was smiling, then he laughed at the memory. His father had put his baby feed into his bottle, but forgot to add the water and left him to feed. When he cried, his father didn't know he had forgotten the water and didn't know what to do with him. This had become a family joke and in time a lever to prove that the father didn't care about his son. But when Antony regressed into this babyhood experience, he saw his father in a different light – as someone who did care but got it wrong!

Advanced hypnosis has two advantages over all other therapies. Once the subject is in hypnosis, you can tap into any memories to find the cause of the problem and discover what were the words that had enough energy to set the faulty programme in motion. Secondly, the subconscious does not have the facility to lie. That is saved for the conscious mind and its logic.

In Antony's case, the regression in hypnosis saved years of conscious therapy. I used all my experience to make sure the change was exceptional and quick. It's not the hypnosis itself that makes the change but the techniques you use when a person is in hypnosis, which is down to the practitioner and their training.

Antony had been putting together a rather interesting workshop himself. It was a very original idea and likely to attract publicity. Before treatment, he didn't seem to attract much enthusiasm and it was a struggle to get anyone to notice him. But now, positive things were happening, hence the journalists and television crew descending on him. Now that he was attracting positiveness in his life, it would follow that he would attract a better type of relationship, too. Instead of someone with stacks of trauma baggage, the type he was usually attracted to, he would hopefully find a more 'together' person, now that his mental cobwebs had been swept away.

A final thought... A recent survey by a magazine published the following information:

1 A British couple can expect their marriage to last nine years. Four out of ten couples divorce.
2 Seventy per cent of divorces are instigated by women.
3 Half the men have not remarried. Thirty-seven per cent wish they were back with their former spouses.

Like many established magazine surveys, no research statistics were published. It's a bit like saying, 'They said...' But it certainly gave me 'food for thought'. I wonder if that's the beginning of a weight problem! Or could it be I'm slim because I'm full of words?!

Useful Addresses

For private clients, couples therapy and 'Learning in Paradise' holidays:

Austin Training Centre
Chesham House
5th floor
150 Regent's Street
London
W1R 5FA

Tel: 0171-465 8440; 0171-637 1320
Fax: 0171-734 4166

Valerie Austin organizes hypnotherapy training courses and stress-reduction courses with her 'Learning in Paradise' holidays in London, Langkawi, Kuala Lumpur, Malaysia, Cyprus, the islands of Tonga, South Pacific and the Caribbean.

To find out more about these, contact the Bluestone Clinic (address above) or the Internet site:

www.paradiselearning.com.

For the official travel agent, quote 'Learning in Paradise' and tel: 01293 537700, fax: 01293 537888; or tel: 0181-569 7192, fax: 0181-560 0815.

Index